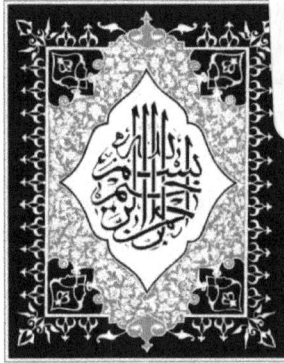

For Every Disease
Allāh Sent Down a Cure

ما أنزل الله داء إلا أنزل له شفاء

mā ʾanzala-llāhu dāʾun ʾillā ʾanzala-llāhu shifāʾ

By Sidi Shaykh Muḥammad Saʿīd al-Jamal ar-Rifāʿī ash-Shādhulī

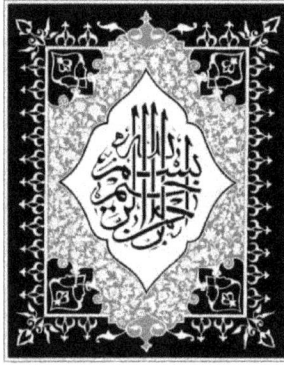

For Every Disease
Allāh Sent Down a Cure

ما أنزل الله داء إلا أنزل له شفاء

mā ʾanzala-llāhu dāʾun ʾillā ʾanzala-llāhu shifāʾ

By Sidi Shaykh Muḥammad Saʿīd al-Jamal ar-Rifāʿī ash-Shādhulī

قال أفرأيتم ما كنتم تعبدون

"And when I am sick, it is He who heals me." (26:75)

بسم الله الرحمٰن الرحيم

الحمد لله رب العالمين

الرحمن الرحيم

مالك يوم الدين

إياك نعبد وإياك نستعين

اهدنـــا الصراط المستقيم

صراط الذين أنعمت عليهم غير المغضوب عليهم ولا الضالين

Cover art: Rahima Wear
Cover design: Amina Stader-Chan

ISBN 978-0-9762150-6-6
© 2011 Sidi Shaykh Muḥammad Saʿīd al-Jamal ar-Rifāʿī ash-Shadhuli
and Shadhiliyya Sufi Center

For information, address the Shadhiliyya Sufi Center
P.O. Box 100 Pope Valley, CA 94567
(707) 965-0700

All material contained within this book is solely informational and is not intended to replace
a licensed healthcare professional's recommendation, diagnosis or treatment plan.

Table of Contents

Introduction 1

The Medicinal Uses of:

Honey 3
Dates 17
    Palm Tree Pollen.. 29
    Date Molasses 30
    Date Seeds.. 31
Bananas 44
Garlic... 50
Onion 57
Black Seed 67
Figs 79
Chamomile... 86
Parsley 88
Date Palm Shoots 89
Lupin.. 89
Strawberries 90
Tamarind.. 91
Arugula... 92
Yellow Carrot 93
Nutmeg... 94
Sycamore.. 95
Fenugreek 96
Chickpeas 97
Common Mallow 98
Carob... 99
Castor Beans 100
Mustard 102
Lettuce.. 104
Ammi 106
Peach 107

Galangal.. 108

Cucumbers 109

Doum 110

Thyme.. 111

Saffron 113

Ginger 115

Olives 116

The Siwak... 117

Barley 119

Fennel 122

Melon 123

Black Tea 124

Date Palm Pollen 126

Tomatoes 128

Sunflower 129

Lentils 130

Juniper 133

Licorice 135

Ambergris 137

Sweetgum... 139

Radish 140

Common Beans... 142

Broad Beans 143

Cinnamon... 144

Cauliflower... 146

Carnation... 147

Stinging Nettle 149

Wheat... 150

Coffee 152

Flax.. 154

Cabbage 157

Coriander... 159

Cumin... 160

White Turnip 161

Lemon 163

Peppermint 169

Al-Ḥijāma (Bleeding Cupping) 171

Gynecology and Childbirth.. 177

Impotence and Sexual Dysfunction 182

The Medicinal Use of Herbs 192

References.. 197

Index 198

Index of Quotes from the Qur'ān.. 216

Index of Quotes from the Ḥadīth.. 217

Introduction

All praise is due to Allāh (﷾) and may the peace and blessings of Allāh (﷾) be upon our most honorable of prophets and messengers (ﷺ), the mercy of Allāh (﷾) to all people, our most honest and promising leader (﷾) and upon all of his family, companions and wives (﷽).

To proceed: the trend that calls for the use of plants and herbs for treating diseases today is in itself a call to return to our Creator's greatness and simplicity (﷾); it is also a call to stay away from the complexities of the various types and forms of chemicals and drugs. This is what world health organizations are seeking to achieve in their research on different diseases that have recently appeared and are spreading. Many scientists and physicians think that these diseases, which did not exist in the past, are a result of the chemical substances used by many patients; these chemical substances are even used by healthy people, who tend to take them regardless of their dangers.

Therefore, many researchers have decided to look more deeply into ancient knowledge in order to include the insights of the past in modern research so that we can take what works for today's generations. To that end, they have researched some herbs and plants unknown to all except our ancestors. As a result, they have created a bond between the original knowledge of the ancients and modern evolution. It is important to note that this is not a call to revert to a primitive mentality or to turn our backs on the scientific research taking place today; it is a call to highlight the significance of the natural resources we still have within our grasp that surround us on this earth, such as herbs, regardless of whether they are used for nutritional supplementation or medication.

We should not underestimate or neglect the triumphs achieved by many physicians working in hospitals equipped with various modern devices (such x-ray machines, etc.) that serve to diagnose a variety of illnesses.

When modern medicines have failed to cure an illness, people search for those who have experience and knowledge in ancient natural remedies. The scientists of the past have passed on the knowledge of what herbs contain in order to heal each and every individual disease. We have authenticated documentation from reliable sources (like the prophets, their wives and their companions ﷺ) that natural remedies have been tried with positive results.

الله

Healing with Honey

I would like to illustrate the use of honey with a story found in some ancient Egyptian scripts and tombs. As discoverers dug in the Egyptian pyramids, they found a child's corpse immersed in honey. The child's corpse did not decay or even rot for 4,500 years. This is evidence of honey's wondrous secrets that, by Allāh's command (ﷻ), were deposited in honey as a cure for every disease. Allāh taʿālā (ﷻ) is truthful, as He says in sūratu-l-nahl:

وأوحى ربك إلى النحل أن اتخذي من الجبال بيوتا
ومن الشجر ومما يعرشون

"And your Lord inspired the bees saying,
'Build yourselves houses in the mountains and in the trees
and in what people construct.'" (16:68)

ثم كلي من كل الثمرات فاسلكي سبل ربك ذللا يخرج من
بطونها شراب مختلف ألوانه فيه شفاء للناس
إن في ذلك لآية لقوم يتفكرون

"'Then feed on all kinds of fruit and follow the ways made easy for you by your Lord.' From their bellies comes a drink of different colors in which there is healing for people. There truly is a sign in this for those who think. (16:68-69)

As mentioned in the Qurʾān, bees act upon revelations from Allāh (ﷻ). These revelations direct them to gather nectar and process it in their bellies, which later emerges as honey from their mouths. This honey carries all of the plants' medical extracts, ready for people to use to cure disease.

On the authority of Ibn ʿAbbās (ﷺ), may Allāh (ﷻ) be pleased with him, the following ḥadīth was transmitted:

The Prophet Muḥammad (ﷺ) says,
"Healing is by three (means): a drink of honey,

cupping and cauterizing with fire;
however, I forbid my nation to use cauterization." (Bukhārī 7:585)

The Prophet Muḥammad (ﷺ), may the peace and blessings of Allāh (ﷻ) upon him, used to drink honey diluted with water on an empty stomach, as mentioned in the book *Zād al-miʿād fī hadī khayr al-ʿibād*.[1] It is even better if honey is drunk with Zamzam water instead of ordinary water; this makes it an inclusive remedy and a beneficial balsam for any disease, as Allāh taʿālā (ﷻ) wills.

Ibn Mājah (ﷺ) mentioned in his sunna taken from Abū Hurayra (ﷺ), may Allāh (ﷻ) be pleased with him, that, "He who licks three drops (of honey) every month will not be infected by great calamities."

Why? It has been proven scientifically, practically and experimentally that bacterial life does not exist in honey, for it contains a high concentration of potassium, which prevents humidity, an important basis for bacterial life.

Honey is full of great mysteries; its wondrous secrets are unbelievable. The sweetness of honey is many times higher than the sweetness of manufactured sugar. There are five to ten types of sugar in honey, including: fructose, dextrose, sucrose, barley sugar and so on. Moreover, honey contains many of the vitamins found in a multi-vitamin, like: A, B_1 (thiamine), B_2 (riboflavin), B_3 (niacin), B_5 (pantothenic acid), B_6 (pyridoxine), B_7 (biotin), B_9 (folic acid), D and K. It has been proven that these vitamins are found in their most powerful and pure forms in honey and they are easily absorbed one hour after consumption, unlike the vitamins found in other foods which are absorbed more weakly and slowly by the body.

---

[1] Ibn Qayyim al-Jawzī (691-751 AH), زاد المعاد في هدي خير العباد. Al-Maktabat-ul-Asriya, 1426 AH (2005 CE), 4,601 pages. This is a book about the Prophet Muḥammad's guidance for Muslims.

Honey also contains iron and minerals, such as iron (Fe), potassium (K), sulfur (S), magnesium (Mg), phosphorus (P), calcium (Ca), iodine (I), sodium (Na), chlorine (Cl), copper (Cu), nickel (Ni), chromium (Cr), lead (Pb), silicon (Si), manganese (Mn), lithium (Li), tin (Sn), aluminum (Al), zinc (Zn) and titanium (Ti). Amazingly, these ingredients are the same components of dirt, from which Allāh taʿālā (﷾) created the human being.

Other valuable components of honey that contribute to human vitality are yeasts and their acids like amylase yeast, invertase yeast, catalase, phosphatase and peroxide. Honey contains a variety of other essential acids, such as: formic acid, lactic acid, citric acid, oxalic acid, pyroglutamic acid, acetic acid and gluconic acid.

Honey also consists of activating and stimulating hormones. Consequently, the antibiotics found in honey protect human beings from different diseases by destroying the most hazardous germs and microbes, inshāʾa-llāh (﷾). The deuterium found in honey, also called heavy hydrogen, is considered an anti-cancer substance, as well as a cure.

The following diseases are treated with honey, inshāʾa-llāh (﷾):

1. Skin Allergies

1. Add some Vaseline and flower oil to a small cup of honey.
2. Apply this mixture to the sensitive skin in the morning and at night.

   - It is better to avoid foods like eggs and mango, for they are known to cause allergies.
   - This remedy is even better when eaten with 1 teaspoon of honey, which enhances the cure, inshāʾa-llāh (﷾).

2. Cosmetic Beautifier for Women and for Facial Clarity

1. Apply honey to your face and leave it on for 15 minutes while allowing your body to relax.

2. Rinse your face with warm water, dry it and apply olive oil.

3. Do this for a week and your face will radiate youthfulness.

   Note: Of course, women should wear a head covering (ḥijāb) so as not to expose their beauty to anyone except their husbands and those who are maḥram.[2]

3. Wounds and Cuts

- Apply some honey to the wound or cut and then cover the area with a bandage. Repeat this treatment every 3 days.

  Note: Avoid wetting the bandage.

  The results will be surprising, for the wound will be healed, leaving no signs of swelling or blisters.

4. Burns

- Mix honey with Vaseline and then apply it to the burned area in the morning and at night until the skin peels. Inshāʾa-llāh (﷾), you will find the skin new, as if it had not been burned at all.

  Note: You can also beat an egg, add 1 teaspoon of honey to this and then apply it to the burned skin daily until it heals.

5. Insomnia

- Add 1 teaspoon of honey to 1 cup of warm milk and drink it 1 hour before bedtime.

---

[2] Men a woman can never marry because of their close relationship to her, like her brother, her father, and so on.

6. Mental Illnesses and Insanity

- Having one's back stung by bees at least once a month helps prevent mental illness.

- Eating a lot of honey and beeswax, as well as rubbing some honey on the back of the head will, inshā'a-llāh (ﷻ), assure a blissful life.

7. Epilepsy

1. Drink about ½ cup of honey on an empty stomach every day.

2. At night before going to sleep, recite from the Qur'ān into a cup of hot water mixed with honey and then drink it.

3. Do this continuously for a week and the illness will be over, inshā'a-llāh (ﷻ).

8. Various Eye Diseases

1. Every morning and night, line your eyes with honey (using it like eyeliner or kohl).

2. Additionally, eat a small teaspoon of honey every day.

9. Gastric Acidity

- Mix 1 cup of milk with 1 teaspoon of honey and use this mixture to swallow a clove of garlic. Do this every day for 5 days.

  Note: Milk with honey can also be drunk as necessary for gastric problems—the more the better.

10. Diarrhea

The following ḥadīth from our Prophet Muḥammad (ﷺ) reminds us of the benefits of honey.

> A man came to the Prophet (ﷺ) and said, "My brother's bowels are loose."
>
> So our Prophet (ﷺ) ordered him to give his brother honey.

The man was in a big hurry. After a short while he returned to the Prophet (ﷺ), claiming that even though his brother ate the honey his condition had worsened.

The Prophet Muḥammad (ﷺ) replied, "Allāh (ﷻ) is truthful and your brother's stomach is false."

This story has been told so that people can learn to be patient when consuming honey as a treatment. The man in the ḥadīth did not wait until the honey was absorbed and thought that it was like water, that it would quench his thirst the moment it was consumed. Honey needs at least 1 hour to be totally consumed by the human digestive system; it is both a food and a remedy that needs time to show its effectiveness. Indeed, as the man returned to check on his brother's condition, he found him totally cured. This proves that honey is an effective remedy.

11. Constipation

- Every morning and evening, dissolve 1 teaspoon of honey in 1 cup of cold milk and drink it. This helps to soften one's stomach and it totally refines it.

12. Vomiting

- Boil some carnation and sweeten it with honey. Drink the mixture before every meal to prevent vomiting and nausea.

13. Perforated Ulcers

1. Put 2 teaspoons of honey in 1 cup of hot milk and add some dried banana peel flour.
2. Take 1 teaspoon of the mixture every morning and evening for a month.

14. Lung Diseases

One Remedy

- Combine radish juice, 1 teaspoon of honey and a warm cup of water. Drink this daily in the morning and at night to help cleanse the lungs.

Another Remedy

- Boil some oliban (Boswellia carteri).[3] Add some honey and then drink it. This is a much stronger and more effective remedy for lung problems, inshā'a-llāh (ﷻ).

15. Halitosis (Bad Breath)

1. Dissolve 2 teaspoons of honey in water.
2. Bring the water to a boil on low heat until it produces a lot of steam. Inhale the steam through the mouth. Repeat this procedure until a change is noticed.

- Chewing beeswax, together with this treatment, assures total disappearance of this disease, inshā'a-llāh ta'ālā.

16. Hoarse Voice

1. Apply the procedure just described for halitosis.
2. In addition, gargle a mixture of water, honey and salt for three days (at most) to put an end to this problem.

17. The Flu

1. Boil water, honey and 1 chopped onion.
2. Inhale its steam before bedtime and take 1 teaspoon of honey after every meal, as well.

18. Herpes

- Boil dill juice with ¼ cup of honey and then preserve it in a jar. Apply this mixture to the sores and, inshā'a-llāh (ﷻ), they will be removed.

---

[3] The primary tree in the genus Boswellia from which frankincense is derived.

19. For Sore Gums and to Strengthen the Teeth

1. Rinse the mouth with a mixture of honey and vinegar every morning and evening.

2. Rub the gums with honey using a siwak.

Note: Honey serves as toothpaste, protecting the teeth from decay and strengthening the gums and teeth.

20. Varicose Veins

1. For various vein diseases and their ulcers, honey is used as a lotion. Apply honey to the affected areas 3 times a day using gentle massage. Repeat this treatment until the problem fades away.

2. Also, have 1 teaspoon of honey after every meal.

21. Chronic Sores and Gangrene

1. Properly mix ½ cup of honey with ½ cup of cod liver oil and apply some of this mixture to the affected area after cleansing it with a sterilizer (honey dissolved in warm water).

2. Cover the area with a bandage and repeat this procedure daily until the skin is healed.

3. It is recommended to drink ½ cup of honey to enhance the remedy.

22. Malignant Tumors

- Use bee glue to bandage the tumors.[4] The tumor must be cleansed every day.

- Of course, we should have 1 teaspoon of honey every morning and every evening before meals.

---

[4] Propolis, or bee glue, is created from resins, balsams and tree saps. The species of honey bees that nest in tree cavities use propolis to seal cracks in the hive.

23. Asthma

1. Combine honey, 1 teaspoon of ginger and 1 teaspoon of vinegar and mix them all together with water.

2. Drink the mixture on an empty stomach every day, and with Allāh's help (﷾) suffering from asthma will cease within weeks.

24. Tuberculosis

1. Mix together equal amounts of rose syrup and honey and drink ½ cup of this mixture every morning and evening.

2. In addition, massage the chest and neck with a mixture of olive oil and honey before bedtime. This should be repeated until Allāh taʿālā (﷾) heals the disease.

25. Strengthening the Heart Muscle

- Boil pomegranate peel in water and then add 1 teaspoon of honey to it. This drink strengthens the heart.

- Taking three drops of royal jelly[5] and a little amber oil is also enough to activate and strengthen the heart.

26. Heart Muscle Inflammation and Arrhythmia

- On a daily basis, drink a cup of cold water sweetened with 2 teaspoons of honey. Continue doing so for a week until the disease is over.

27. Heart Pressure

- Have 1 teaspoon of honey after every meal for a month.

- Drink 1 cup of carrot juice or wheatgrass juice and the heart will heal inshāʾa-llāh (﷾).

28. Inflammation of the Mouth and Tongue Diseases

- Add 1 teaspoon of honey to ½ cup hot water and gargle with it 3 times a day. This will heal the disease in days, inshāʾa-llāh (﷾).

---

[5] Food for the queen bee and the larvae who may become queen.

29. Ear Diseases and Pain

- Dissolve some honey in water and then mix with little salt. Drop into the infected ear before bedtime every day.

30. Rheumatism (Joint and/or Connective Tissue Pain)

- Add honey and 1 teaspoon of black seed to 1 cup of warm water and drink.

- One can also massage the affected area with a mixture comprised of equal amounts of black seed oil, olive oil, and eucalyptus oil. Add some honey to the mixture, apply it to the afflicted area and then wrap it with a piece of wool in a way that does not add pressure.

- It is also evident that beestings on the painful organ or joint will eliminate rheumatism. The area should be rubbed with honey afterward.

31. Ascites

1. Drink a mixture of boiled oliban and honey every morning and evening.

2. Rub some of the mixture about 1 inch above and below the navel. This is tested method for completely curing ascites. It is important to rely on oats, honey and whole wheat bread as your main foods for 3 days afterward.

32. Alopecia from Infection (hair loss)

1. Shave and sterilize the infected area properly until it begins to rend.

2. Rub the infected area with bee venom and bandage it. This bandage should be changed every day at the same hour for 1 week.

33. Calluses

1. Heat some royal jelly and smear it on the callus.

2. Then tie it properly and leave it alone for three days until the callus totally drops off.

34. Kidney Stones / Renal Colic

1. Cook some leaves of the wild hibiscus flower and strain them well, saving the liquid.
2. Then add 3 teaspoons of honey and 1 teaspoon of butter made from cow's milk to the hibiscus tea.
3. Mix it properly and drink a cup of this mixture when the renal colic begins.
4. This should be repeated for 1 week until the kidney stones are totally dissolved.

35. Liver Diseases

1. Grind oak bark finely into a powder and mix 1 teaspoon of it with ½ cup of honey.
2. This mixture should be eaten on an empty stomach constantly and daily for 1 month.

36. To Provide Strength, Vitality and Youthfulness

- Behold this golden advice: do not let a day pass by without having 1 teaspoon of honey as if it were water; consider it a habit for the rest of your life. Ibn Sīnā (ﷺ) says, "If you intend to preserve your youth, eat honey."[6]

- You can also boil some walnut leaves, strain them properly and then add some honey to them. This should be drunk as a tea every day. This is a very powerful energizer.

---

[6] Abū ʿAlī al-Ḥusayn ibn ʿAbd Allāh ibn Sīnā (ﷺ) (980-1037 C.E.) was a famous scholar who wrote almost 450 treatises on a wide range of subjects, many of which concentrate on philosophy and medicine.

As one of the knowledgeable men says:

> Moderation in everything is life's balance.
> The secret of strength and health
> is in the good things created for us.
> The secret of mental health is in virtual
> moralities.
> The sun, open air and exercise
> are the best protection from illness and drugs.

> Prefer to eat everything
> Allāh (﷾) has created fresh and ripe,
> and beware of chemical medicines
> that only demolish what you have built.
>
> Finally, watch out for three deadly things:
> staying awake at night, lack of sleep and
> anxiety.

38. Gynecology and Labor

- Drinking ½ cup honey when contractions begin during labor will help to smooth the progress of a woman's labor, inshā'a-llāh (﷾). It is important for a woman to continue to eat honey with wheat bread after childbirth.

- To help reduce the pain and discomfort of menopause, a woman can drink a cup of boiled fenugreek with some honey every morning and evening. It is also advised to clean the vagina with a mixture of warm water and honey, which will be quite relieving for menopausal women.

39. Reproductive Improvement

1. Heat the juice of 3 onions with the same amount of honey on low heat until the honey's foam dissolves. This can be stored for several uses.

2. One teaspoon of this mixture can be taken after lunch on a daily basis.

3. To further enhance this remedy, one can add some black seed or radish seed and eat it like jam; even an elderly man will notice the difference.

40. Infertility

1. Eat some royal jelly the moment you extract it from a beehive and then follow this with a mixture of milk and about 3 mg. rhinoceros horn filings.[7]

2. Do this for a month and, inshā'a-llāh (ﷻ), you will be granted children.

41. Cancer

1. Immediately after removing about 100 mg. of royal jelly from a beehive, eat it with 1 cup of honey along with its wax. Do this every week.

2. After eating the royal jelly and wax, receive a whole body massage that uses honey and black seed. Wash the honey and black seed off with warm water after 1 hour.

3. Drink a mixture of honey and ground black seed in 1 cup of carrot juice daily.

42. Leprosy and Vitiligo[8]

- A daily application of honey with some ammonia on the affected areas will clear these skin diseases.

---

[7] This refers to pieces of rhinoceros horn that have naturally broken off of the animal. This remedy should be only used as a last resort.

[8] Vitiligo is a skin condition in which there is a loss of pigment from areas of skin, resulting in irregular white patches that feel like normal skin.

43. Poisoning/Toxicity

1. Add 1 teaspoon of sesame oil to 1 cup of honey and drink the mixture every morning and evening.

2. Also, add some honey and several drops of amber oil to a hot cup of milk. Drink this mixture for three days and do not eat meat during that time.

44. Prostatitis

1. Eat about 50 mg. of royal jelly daily, immediately after extracting it from a beehive.

2. Wash the infected area with a mixture of warm water and honey every evening for a month.

Heal Yourself With Dates

The date palm tree is mentioned twenty times in the Holy Qur'ān. Two examples are:

ومن النخل من طلعها قنوان دانية

"From the date palm come clusters of low-hanging dates..." (6:99)

فيها فاكهة والنخل ذات الأكمام

"Within it are fruits and date palm trees with sheathed clusters (of dates)." (55:11)

Dates in the Sunna

On the authority of Amīr bin Sa'd bin Abū Waqqās (﷽) the Prophet Muḥammad (﷽), may the peace and blessings of Allāh (﷽) upon him, said:

> He who eats seven dates as he awakens,
> no poison or spell will harm him that day. (Muslim 23:5081)

Ibn Nawāwi (﷽) says, "The intrinsic worth and wisdom behind eating dates directly after waking up in the morning and preferring the Medina dates over other dates, in addition to the number seven, are yet unknown to people. Nevertheless, we should believe and have faith in their virtues."

Again, Abū Hurayra (﷽), may Allāh (﷽) be pleased with him, said:

> The Prophet Muḥammad (﷽) said:
> "Dates are from Paradise and contain a cure for poison;
> truffles are a kind of manna and their juice is a medicine for the eye." (Tirmidhi 1127)

'Ā'isha (﷽), may Allāh (﷽) be pleased with her, narrated:

> The Prophet Muḥammad (﷽) said, "'Ā'isha, a home without dates has within it a hungry family."
> He repeated this two or three times. (Muslim 23:5079)

The Prophet Muḥammad (ﷺ), may the peace and blessings of Allāh (﷽) upon him and his family (ﷺ), used to smear dates on the lips of newborns in Medina and pray for their blessings. Abū Mūsā said:

> I brought my newborn son to the Prophet (ﷺ) and He named him Ibrāhīm and then he smeared his lips (palate) with his dates. (Muslim 25:5343)

ʿAbdullāh bin Omar (ﷺ) said:

> The Prophet (ﷺ) said, "Among the trees, there is a tree,
> the leaves of which do not fall
> and (in this way) is like a Muslim. Tell me the name of that tree."
>
> Everybody started thinking about the trees in the desert.
> And I thought of the date palm tree but felt shy to answer.
> The others then asked, "What is that tree, oh Messenger of Allāh
> (﷽)?" He replied, "It is the date-palm tree." (Bukhārī 3:58)

The Prophet Muḥammad (ﷺ), may the peace and blessing of Allāh (﷽) upon him, said:

> Feed your wives dates during their nifās,[9]
> for she who eats dates during her nifās produces a wise child.
>
> Dates were Maryam's food (ﷺ) when she gave birth to ʿĪsā (Jesus)
> (ﷺ). If Allāh taʿālā (﷽) had a better food for her, He would have fed
> her with it.

The Prophet Muḥammad (ﷺ), may the peace and blessings of Allāh (﷽) upon him, said as well:

> Break your fast by eating dates.
> If you do not have dates, then drink water, for it is purifying.
> (Abū Dāwūd 13:2348)

---

[9] Time of bleeding after childbirth.

Anas ibn Malik (▦), may Allāh (▦) be pleased with him, said:

> The Prophet Muḥammad (▦) used to break his fast before praying
> with some fresh dates; but if there were no fresh dates,
> he had a few dry dates and if there were no dry dates,
> he took some mouthfuls of water. (Abū Dāwūd 13:2349)

The Prophet Muḥammad said:

> The highest date has the best cure.

> The best dates are the Burni dates (from Medina) which prevent
> disease and have no disease in them.

In another version Abū Hurayra (▦) quotes:

> Burni Dates are a remedy that do not bear a malady.

Allāh taʿālā (▦) says:

$$والنخل باسقات لها طلع نضيد$$

"And tall palm trees laden with clusters of dates." (50:10)

These are to emphasize the importance of dates that come from a good tree.

$$شجرة طيبة أصلها ثابت وفرعها في السماء$$
$$تؤتي أكلها كل حين بإذن ربها$$

"A good tree whose root is firm and whose branches are high in the sky,
yielding constant fruit by its Lord's leave." (14:24-25)

Dates are the first food to enter the baby's stomach after its mother's milk and they are the first food fasting Muslims have after a long day without food. Allāh (▦) ordered Maryam (▦) to shake the date palm's trunk so that many ripe and pure dates would drop for her sustenance and protection.

Dates and Birth

Allāh taʿālā (ﷻ) says:

وهزي إليك بجذع النخلة تساقط عليك رطبا جنيا

فكلي واشربي وقري عينا فإما ترين من البشر أحدا فقولي إني

نذرت للرحمن صوما فلن أكلم اليوم إنسيا

"And, if you shake the trunk of the palm tree toward you,
it will deliver fresh ripe dates to you,
so eat, drink and be glad and say to anyone you may see,
'I have vowed to the Lord of Mercy to abstain from conversation
and I will not talk to anyone today.'" (19:25-26)

The purpose of eating dates at the beginning of a meal after fasting is revealed in the following narration by Anas ibn Malik (ﷺ):

> The Prophet Muḥammad (ﷺ) used to break his fast before praying
> with some fresh dates; but if there were no fresh dates,
> he had a few dry dates and if there were no dry dates,
> he took some mouthfuls of water. (Abū Dāwūd 13:2349)

Salmān bin ʿAmr (ﷺ) said:

> The Prophet Muḥammad (ﷺ) said, "When one of you is fasting,
> you should break your fast with dates; but if you cannot get any,
> then (you should break your fast) with water,
> for water is purifying." (Abū Dāwūd 13:2348)

The Prophet Muḥammad, may the peace and blessings of Allāh (ﷻ) be upon him, has specifically chosen this food for many reasons. Eating different kinds of dates provides the body with large amounts of carbohydrates in a short amount of time, especially after fasting when the stomach and intestines are empty and ready to work and quickly absorb nutrition. Dates contain a relatively high percentage of humidity.

Additionally, dates are two-thirds carbohydrates in their simple structure, which is easily broken down in the first digestive cycle. This reduces the level of sugar in the blood within a short period of time. The intestines absorb the water and sugar contained in dates in less than five minutes, which quenches the fasting person's thirst and reduces any symptoms of sugar loss. A person who has fasted and immediately fills his stomach with different types of food and drink needs 3-4 hours for his digestive system to absorb the sugar from his meal.

Another fact: dates contain a high proportion of cellulosic fibers that benefit fasting people. These fibers act as sponges, sucking up the water in the intestines, which results in a natural softening of the feces. As a result, fasting people will not suffer from constipation. Because there is a reduced amount of food consumed, the amount of waste in the gut is also reduced, thus preventing any health complications like digestive disorders or hemorrhoids during fasting.

In this way, the prophetic wisdom of breaking one's fast with dates for the simple carbohydrates is revealed.

Microbes Do Not Survive in Dates
The Prophet Muḥammad (ﷺ), may the peace and blessings of Allāh (﷼) be upon him, said, "The best dates are the Burni dates (from Medina), which prevent disease and have no diseases in them."

Truly, dates do not carry diseases, for microorganisms cannot live in them.

An experiment was held to examine this fact. Fresh dates were contaminated with three different types of cholera germs at levels 100-1000 times greater than what was evident in cholera patients' excrement. These germs did not survive for more than three days, proving that if dates are exposed to severe contamination, they will be non-infectious and will remain edible. Studies indicate that dates have a layer of tannins which provide protection from parasites; tannins cause decadent spots on the surface when ripe.

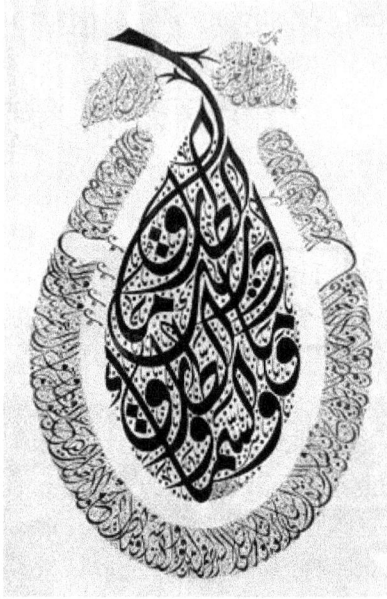

Dates Protect Us from Cancer

Another great feature of dates is that they are rich in magnesium, which is a known anti-cancer substance. Rarely can you find a Bedouin with cancer who relies on dates as a primary food.

Rubbing Dates on the Lips of Newborns (Tahnik)

Taḥnīk is a medical miracle of our Prophet Muḥammad (ﷺ), may the peace and blessings of Allāh (﷾) be upon him. The wisdom behind it was not revealed until recently. Today, the critical period of time between a child's birth and when he or she begins to breastfeed is treated almost as if it were irrelevant; it has not been given the attention it requires.

However, the Prophet Muḥammad (ﷺ), may the peace and blessings of Allāh (﷾) be upon him, blessed newborns by rubbing dates on their lips, knowing that dates contain a sufficient amount of carbohydrates that can be easily absorbed into the babies' veins. This helps the baby maintain a normal blood sugar level, and it can even raise low blood sugar until the baby learns to breastfeed normally.

The Benefits of Dates in Curing Disease

1. Constipation

- It is a fact that dates contain a high percentage of fructose, which is known to be quite beneficial for the intestines. Normal peristalsis helps prevent constipation.

2. Poisoning

The Prophet Muḥammad (ﷺ) said, "Ripe dates are from Paradise and they contain the cure for every poison."

- He recommends eating 7 dates in the morning, preferably, Medina dates.

- He also recommends pressing them on stings, bites or pain caused by any type of poisonous creature.

3. Eye Diseases

1. Roast date pits after washing them properly and then grind them like coffee beans until they are a smooth paste.

2. Mix equal amounts of the ground date pits and antimony (kohl).

3. Use this mixture to line the eyes to protect them from diseases and to serve as eyeliner.

4. Rheumatism

- Experiments have proven that dates are the source of some medicines that doctors prescribe for rheumatic patients.

5. Lung Diseases

1. Take 7 dates and weigh them.

2. Add the same amount (in weight) of raisins, jujube (red dates) and figs.

3. Cook all ingredients in 1 liter of water until the mixture is reduced to half of its original quantity.

4. Mash the mixture and then strain it, saving the liquid.

5. Drink ½ cup of the liquid before every meal.

6. Asthma

1. Boil some hyssop and then add about ½ cup date molasses to the hyssop.

2. Drink some of this mixture every morning and evening.

• Avoid eating allergy-causing foods such as eggs, fish and mango.

7. To Provide Strength, Vitality and Youthfulness

1. Remove the pits of 7 dates and mix them with crushed nuts (i.e. pine seeds, hazelnuts or almonds) in addition to 1 teaspoon of indigenous margarine.

2. This blend should be eaten daily on an empty stomach and followed with a warm drink of boiled chamomile tea.

• This recipe helps strengthen the heart and boosts the nerves.

8. Reproductive Improvement

1. Take a handful of pressed dates and add 7 yolks and 1 teaspoon of indigenous margarine.

2. Stir together and cook until the mixture becomes smooth.

• This should be eaten with whole wheat bread for breakfast and then followed by 1 cup of milk or carrot juice.

9. For the Treatment of Inactivity and Laziness

• One hundred grams of dates contain 40-72 grams of phosphorus. Phosphorus activates brain cells, as well as the pineal gland, which activates the human brain and improves intelligence. Phosphorus is also needed to nourish and refresh the noble regions of the brain.

- Moreover, 100 grams of dates consists of 80-100 IUs of vitamin A, known to be essential for calming the nervous system. Therefore, it allows for more concentrated thinking without adding stress.

10. Heart Disease

- Dates are the finest remedy. They help strengthen the human body and support its systems. They are rich in phosphors and sulfurs, which melt accumulated fats and soften the arteries.

- In addition, dates enhance the heart muscles, for they contain choline, a substance known to eliminate carditis and arteritides.[10]

- The high proportion of phosphorus in dates helps purify the blood, which eventually creates a healthier and happier life.

11. To Prevent Kidney Failure

- Continuous consumption of dates generates more urine and cleanses the urinary tract, which prevents the formation of kidney stones and excessive minerals.

- Dates eliminate various types of kidney inflammation and infection. They heat up the kidneys, which helps protect them from kidney failure, inshā'a-llāh (ﷻ). The effectiveness of dates lies not only in the carbohydrates and phosphorus they contain, but they also consist of colloidal and gluten substances that prevent the scraping of the renal tubes and the kidneys.

- Such protection is enhanced, for dates also contain essential vitamins (i.e. B_1, B_2, etc.), which are considered fortifiers for the nerves and they eliminate infection.

---

[10] Inflammation and infection of the heart and arteries

12. Anemia

- Given the fact that dates contain iron, they are the best remedy for iron-deficiency anemia.

13. Infertility

1. Take about 1 cup of ground palm acacia and mix it with 1 kg. of honey.

2. After every breakfast and dinner, both the husband and wife should take 1 teaspoon of this mixture.

3. The wife should also use this remedy as a vaginal suppository before bedtime on a daily basis.

14. Gastric Acid

1. Dates have alkaline minerals, which make them suitable for preventing acidity of the stomach or blood.

2. They also help in preventing gastric ulcers and they minimize the possibility of developing colon cancer.

3. These minerals prevent the production of stones, both in the kidneys and the gallbladder.

15. Dizziness

- Swallow 7 ripe dates one after another on an empty stomach. This should be done daily until the dizziness fades away.

16. Night Blindness

1. The best remedy is to eat dates as much as possible, in addition to cleansing the eyes with palm fronds boiled in water.

2. This mixture helps cleanse sores on the eyes, washes off dirt that harms the eyes, and clears off blurriness.

17. Psoriasis

1. Burn some palm fronds until they turn into ashes.

2. Combine 1 cup of the ash with 1 kg. of honey.

3. Apply the mixture to the infected areas.

- Also, eat many dates for their zinc content, which is appropriate for this disease.

18. Bleeding Hemorrhoids

- Mix ½ cup of the juice from mussels with ½ teaspoon of ground tannins together and drink it after every breakfast and dinner.

19. Mental Illnesses

1. Peel off the covering of a palm trunk and wash the peel carefully.

2. Boil it in water, strain it and then drink the water like a tea. Of course, you can sweeten it with some sugar cane.

3. This should be repeated every morning and evening.

The Medicinal Use of Palm Tree Pollen

(Palm Heart)

1. Asthma
   - Mix palm tree pollen with some date molasses and eat it as a remedy to vanquish sensitivity in the pulmonary system, which relieves asthma.

2. Gastric Bleeding
   - Eat some pollen and drink chamomile tea every day on an empty stomach.
   - Palm heart is one of the most powerful remedies for treating gastric diseases.

3. Whooping Cough
   1. Eat some palm pollen and drink date molasses.
   2. Rub the chest with palm oil before going to sleep and, inshā'a-llāh (﷽), the coughing will end.

4. Diarrhea
   1. Palm heart serves multiple purposes: it relaxes intestinal contractions while cleansing and sterilizing, which makes it a most effective remedy for diarrhea.

5. Wound Healing and Sores
   2. Mince the pollen and mix it together with honey and henna, and then you will have one of the most powerful ointments for treating sores, cuts and wounds.

The Medicinal Use of Date Molasses

(Date Honey or Juice)

1. **Respiratory Diseases**

    1. Use for treating respiratory maladies such as cough. It expels sputum and mucus trapped in the respiratory system while enhancing it. To achieve this effect, simply drink about ½ cup of date molasses daily on an empty stomach.

    2. Then, swallow 1 chopped clove of garlic and drink some hot water. This helps to expel the sputum and put an end to the coughing, in addition to fortifying the respiratory system.

    3. It works because date palm molasses contains two of the most powerful minerals: iron and copper, which are known to be very effective in curing respiratory diseases.

2. **Arrhythmia**[11]

    4. Drink ½ cup of date molasses every day and afterward eat any type of fruit desired.

---

[11] Abnormal electrical activity in the heart.

The Medicinal Use of Date Seeds

1. **Diabetes**
    1. Roast the date seeds as you would roast coffee beans.
    2. Grind the roasted seeds and mix them with date molasses.
    3. This should be eaten every morning and evening; do not add any sugar to it.

2. **Arteriosclerosis**[12]
    1. Roast the date seeds as you would roast coffee beans.
    2. Grind the roasted seeds and mix them with date molasses.
    3. Eat this mixture with whole wheat bread for breakfast every morning. Swallow 1 clove of garlic, as well, with this meal.

---

[12] Hardening of the arteries.

The Hidden Secrets and Mysteries of Dates

An American commercial once showed a physician saying, "Have two dates and call me in the morning. Be sure to let me know how well they eliminated your constipation." If American physicians treat their patients suffering from constipation with dates, then why don't we (and physicians in the Arabian Peninsula, known to be the birthplace of dates since ancient times) advise our own patients to eat dates?

"Many people suffer from hemorrhoids and one of the common causes is constipation," is a quote from the Science Department at the University of California (1991). The best way to avoid hemorrhoids is to avoid constipation. Therefore, drink a lot of water and eat foods rich in fiber, such as vegetables and fruits.

Eating dates is, without a doubt, quite helpful in eliminating constipation. In this way, you can avoid having hemorrhoids. Dates are rich in dietary fiber; in every 100 grams of dates there are 8.5 grams of fiber.

American and European researchers recommend increasing your daily consumption of dietary fiber to 20-30 grams.

Scientists have recently focused their interest on the benefits of dietary fiber. Foods rich in fiber help people lose excessive weight while protecting them from colorectal cancer, splenic flexure syndrome (colon spasm), colon infections and ulcers, and coronary artery disease.

Dates and Hypertension

Hypertension is one of the most common diseases today. It has been given a great deal of attention, for it is the most important modifiable risk factor that can help prevent stroke, kidney disease and heart attacks. Many studies in this field point out that foods rich in potassium can both prevent and cure hypertension.

Nutritionists, thus, advise hypertension patients to consume foods rich in potassium and to avoid salty foods.

Some claim that lack of magnesium increases the risk for hypertension. When examining the amount of sodium in dates, one finds that in every 100 grams of dates there are only about 5 milligrams of sodium. This is a very small proportion compared to the amount of salt found in other foods (most people consume 3-6 grams daily). So dates are virtually salt-free.

As I will elaborate later, dates are rich in potassium and magnesium, which makes them the ideal remedy for hypertension.

The Composition of Dates
Dates are a rich source of carbohydrates and dietary fiber. Recent scientific research and the World Health Organization (WHO), acknowledge dates as one of the richest foods in carbohydrates and dietary fiber that is fat-free.

Every 100 grams of dates (10-12 dates) contain approximately 248-297 calories; this varies according to the type and ripeness of the date. This is almost ½ the calories found in a chocolate bar. In addition, dates are the richest fruit in vitamins A, B$_1$ (thiamine), B$_2$ (riboflavin), B$_3$ (niacin), and C.

Calories	248 cal.
Carbohydrates	63.9 gr.
Dietary Fiber	8.7 gr.
Protein	2 gr.
Fat	very low
Sodium	5 ml.
Potassium	750 ml.
Calcium	68 ml.
Magnesium	59 ml.
Phosphorus	64 ml.
Iron	1.6 ml.
Copper	.21 ml.

The Date Palm and Potassium
Eating 100 grams of dates a day (about 10-12 dates) guarantees that at least half of your body's daily needs for potassium will be met. Your body needs 1800-5600

milligrams of potassium per day and in 100 grams of dates there are 750 milligrams of potassium.

Potassium is essential for ensuring the proper functioning of the heart, the muscles and the nervous system, and it also helps maintain normal blood sugar levels.

Lack of potassium results in muscle fatigue, loss of appetite, weariness, poor concentration, laziness, constipation, arrhythmia and muscle spasms. In this case, lack of potassium would be treated in a hospital by prescribing medications such as Lasix (Furosemid), used in the treatment of congestive heart failure and edema, in order to generate more urine to maintain a close-to-normal level of potassium. Physicians normally recommend eating foods rich in potassium, such as tomatoes, bananas, potatoes, dates, bran, nuts and oranges.

Dates and Iron

According to the chart on page 33, consuming 100 grams of dates provides the human body with one-sixth of its daily recommended iron. Anemia is considered one of the common nutrition-based problems in America and Europe. According to the University of California's research, 15% of American women have iron deficiency and half of the third world population is anemic. Iron deficiency, if left untreated, leads to anemia, which is a problem for many women, especially during pregnancy.

Dates and Magnesium

One hundred grams of dates provide the human body with one-fifth of its daily recommended dose of magnesium. This ingredient is essential, for it has a fundamental role in creating energy and in cell regeneration. It is an important mineral because it carries nerve impulses to different part of the human body.

Lack of magnesium results in the following: fatigue, general weakness, muscle spasms and fibrillation. It some cases, it may also cause irritation and annoyance. It can lead to ventricular tachycardia, which is a very dangerous illness.[13]

It has been found that 20% of those who take Digoxin, a medicine used to treat various heart conditions, suffer from lack of magnesium.

Dates and Niacin (Vitamin B₃)

Consuming 100 grams of dates provides one-sixth of the recommended daily dose of niacin. Chronic deficiency in this vitamin can lead to a dangerous disease called pellagra. Pellagra is characterized by diarrhea, dermatitis, dementia and death (the four Ds).

Ripe Dates and Labor

Some writers point out that eating ripe dates when a woman is about to go through labor helps the uterus to expand. Dr. Mustafa Mahmud, in his article published in the magazine *Al-ʿIlm wa-l-imān* (Science and Faith Magazine) states, "The latest scientific research about ripe dates has found that they consist of a substance that relieves birth contractions and prevents postnatal bleeding." So, that was Allāh taʿālā's (ﷻ) purpose in telling Maryam (ؤ) to eat ripe dates during and after her labor. Allāh (ﷻ) says:

وهزي إليك بجذع النخلة تساقط عليك رطبا جنيا

"And, if you shake the trunk of the palm tree toward you,
it will deliver fresh ripe dates to you." (19:25)

Al-Baydawī (ؤ) interpreted Maryam's situation (ؤ) and the offering of dates as follows:

> It is said that it was a dry palm with neither top nor fruit. It was winter. She (Maryam) (ؤ) shook it and Allāh taʿālā (ﷻ) created ripe dates for her. She was worthy of this blessing, for she was innocent and pure. She, who had never committed anything

---

[13] A condition in which the resting heart rate exceeds the normal range.

ḥarām (forbidden), was watched over by Him, who is able to produce ripe dates from a dry palm in the winter and is able to impregnate her without a man.

Ar-Rabīʿ bin Haytham (ﷺ) said:

> There is no better remedy I can think of
> for a woman in the post-partum period
> other than ripe dates, due to this Prophetic saying,
> "If Allāh ta'ālā (ﷻ) knew of a better food for Her,
> He would have fed it to Maryam (ﷺ)."

One of the Prophet Muḥammad's (ﷺ) most wonderful sayings about dates is:

> "'Ā'isha, a home without dates has within it a hungry family." He repeated this two or three times. (Muslim 23:5079)

The Prophet Muḥammad (ﷺ), may the peace and blessings of Allāh (ﷻ) be upon him, also said:

> He who eats seven dates as he awakens,
> no poison or spell will harm him that day. (Muslim 23:5081)

Postpartum Period

Dates provide us with the thermal energy our bodies need within a short period of time. Therefore, dates are recommended by physicians to facilitate labor, stop postnatal bleeding and restore the uterus to its natural state.

Rest assured, the date palm provides excellent and vital nutrition for the human body because it has indispensable ingredients that help us maintain the best of health. Some of these components assist in the human being's healthy growth, for they produce new cells and repair those that are damaged. Other components protect the body from disease and help produce antibiotics or enzymes and necessary yeasts for crucial biological processes. Additionally, other components in dates prevent parasites and chronic diseases from harming the body, such as cancer.

By analyzing a date, many facts are gleaned. The fleshy tissue of the date consists of 13-15% water, 70-78% carbohydrates, 2.5% fat, 1.9-2% protein, 10% dietary fiber and 1.5% cinder.[14] Also, in every 100 grams of dates there are 65 milligrams of calcium, 72 milligrams of phosphorus and 5.1 milligrams of iron. Dates are a good source of vitamins A, B and C. There is much research proving that dates contain various essential acids and minerals.

As for the hard tissue of the date, the core or the seed, it comprises approximately 10-20% of the weight of a date. Analysis confirms that it contains 6.5% water, 62.5% carbohydrates, 8.5% fat, 5.5% protein, 16% dietary fiber and 1.5% cinder. It contains various acids, as well; the hard tissue is 7% sulfuric acid, 24% lauric acid, .5% chamber acid, 9.3% myristic acid, 10% palmitic acid, 25% oleic and linoleic acids and 3.2% citric acid. Date seed oil is higher quality than cotton seed oil and thus is superior for human usage. Also, date seeds are ground and used as feed for livestock because of their rich protein content.

The date palm is considered the finest plant the human being has ever known. It is believed to originate in the Persian Gulf and the surrounding area; its plantations are still widely spread throughout Iraq, Iran and the Arabian Peninsula. Date palms also exist on the Mediterranean coast where the climate is relatively cool and, therefore, they are not very common there. However, date palms spread and increase along the southern sides, as in Aswan, where date palm plantations are successfully developing, especially at the oasis located in the Libyan deserts and Sinna, The Lake, al-Farafira, al-Dakhila and al-Kharija in the Arab Republic of Egypt.

---

[14] Cinder is rock made primarily of volcanic substances that is very porous and low-density.

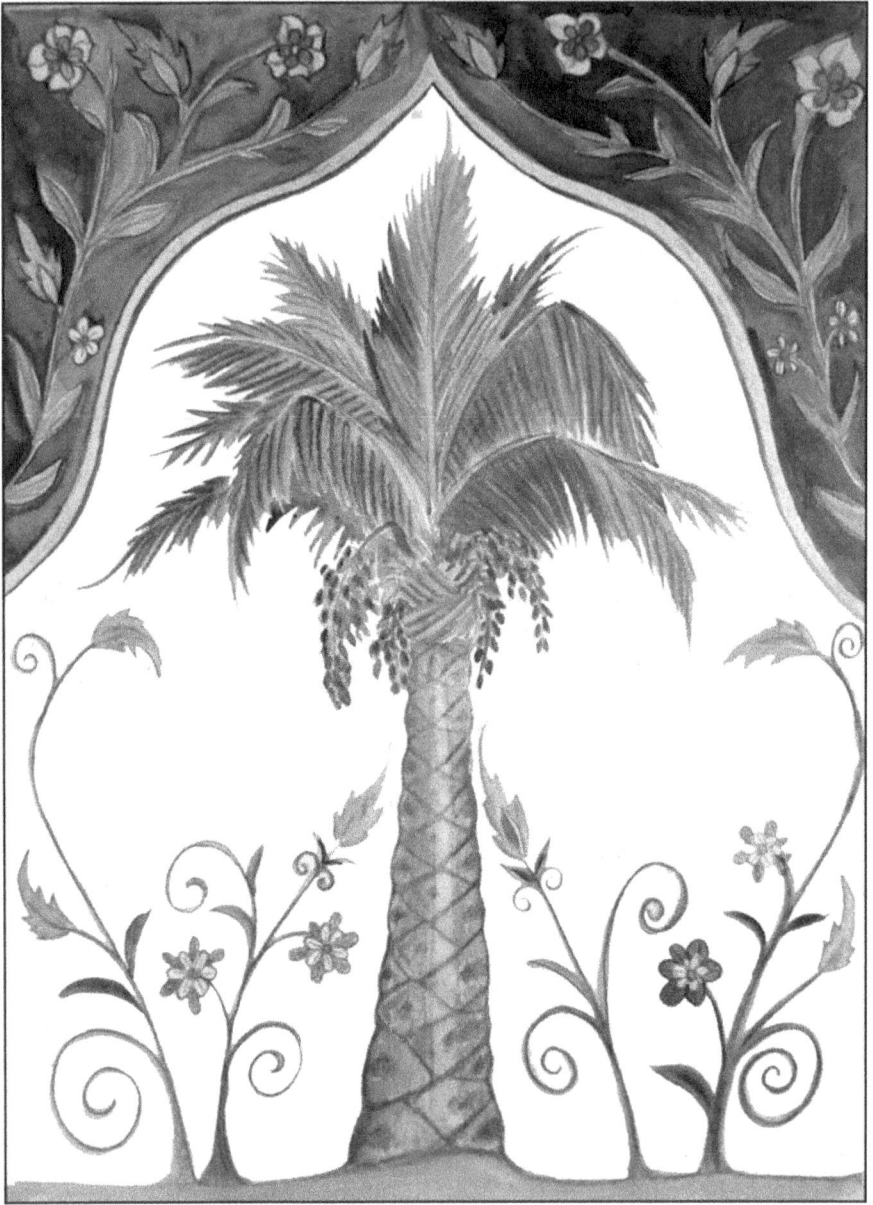

Artwork by Huda al-Jamal

The Date Palm Comes in 3 Types

1. **Dried (stale) dates,** which we name "Tamr." This date is low in humidity and high in carbohydrates. This type of date is easily preserved and if left for more time in the sun, it gets very dry and is edible for a very long time. They are called, "A'fiya" in Egypt. They are extremely dry and if they are put in water, they become soft and hydrated. The most popular dates of this type are: Ibrimi, Barakawi (from Sudan), Gandela, Garguda, Bartmuda and Dijna.

2. **Half-dry dates** are neither dry nor ripe. They are called "Mao" and they, too, can be preserved in natural ways for a very long time. Some dates of this type are: Ameri (also called "the visitor's date," and they are from Iraq) and Ajlani.

3. **Wet dates** are the third type of date. These are difficult to dry using natural methods. These dates are eaten immediately after harvested while they are ripe and juicy.

Dates: Integrated Food and Healing Remedy

Dates contain carbohydrates and starches, which make them easily absorbed by the human digestive system. These carbohydrates exist in the form of glucose, which is the body's main source of energy. More glucose leads to increased circulation, supports the proper functioning of the liver, and provides the body with vitality. In addition, carbohydrates take part in cell construction and they help create antibiotics for the immune system. They support the processing of fats and proteins and they also contain fats essential for the human body. Excessive carbohydrates, in the end, are stored in the liver for future use.

Rich in Vitamins, Minerals and Salts

Dates contain vitamin A, which strengthens vision, especially night vision. This vitamin does not go through the retina, but it plays an important role in the development of bones and teeth. It is involved in body growth and it grants the skin a youthful look. Dates contain other vitamins, such as the B vitamins, that enhance the nervous system and the body's growth. Also, dates contain vitamin C, which helps heal wounds and stop bleeding, and it also protects the gums.

Dates also contain magnesium, which calms the nervous system and is involved in the building of bones, teeth and muscle. Magnesium assists in cell regeneration and it activates necessary yeasts and their biological processes.

The potassium in dates has a tranquilizing effect and it contributes to the proper functioning of the muscles and the transmission of messages throughout the nervous system. Potassium helps maintain cell balance and it organizes the heart's work, as well.

As for the calcium found in dates, it is responsible for the human skeleton. It helps in the production of milk, it prevents nerve excitability and spasms, it clots the blood when there is a wound and it stops bleeding. It is very important for the proper functioning of the heart.

The date, with all of its components, calms the human body and minimizes irritability and nervousness. Due to the fact that dates contain chlorine and sodium, the body's most important minerals, dates help the body and many of its systems attain proper balance.

In addition, zinc, another essential ingredient, is involved in the composition of many fundamental activities, such as human growth, skin protection, wound healing and the reinforcement of the immune system. Copper deals with certain types of anemia and helps in the construction of essential elements in the body. Finally, iron is primary in preventing anemia. Thus, one should consistently consume dates in order to receive all that is necessary for a healthy life, inshā'a-llāh (ﷻ).

During childbirth, the uterus contracts with frequency and intensity and its muscles require great energy and strength to work properly. The most suitable food, in this case, is the one that is the most easily digested, quickly absorbed and nutritious. The carbohydrates in dates, especially the ripe ones, meet these requirements precisely. Ripe dates, in particular, consist of substances similar to oxytocin, the hormone that initiates the uterus's contractions and helps the nerves to rest during labor. Oxytocin promotes relaxation and also stops bleeding. In this way, dates help to balance labor by enhancing weak contractions and easing strong ones.

A pregnant woman who has relied upon ripe dates before her child's birth directly transforms their essential components and delivers them to the fetus through the placenta. A mother who also relies upon ripe dates after her child's birth will have no difficulties generating milk for her baby. Her milk will be very rich with various important and beneficial nutrients. The infant will have the opportunity to drink the most nutritious milk possible, in addition to experiencing greater tranquility. This baby will be the calmest baby you have ever seen! Therefore, this saying is proven to be true, "She who eats ripe dates during her nifās will be granted a calm child." Dates and motherhood are inseparable, as in the saying, "I have nothing better to offer women than ripe dates."

Dates ease irritated teeth and relieve coughing. Dates are very useful for treating mental diseases, for they contain elements that calm and relax the human body. They are light on the digestive system and they lessen vomiting, as well as facilitating bowel movements. The one who regularly eats dates will experience neither constipation nor diarrhea, for dates contain cellulose and pectin. In addition, dates help clarify the leftovers from salts and carbohydrates in the ends of the intestines and the stomach.

Some antibacterial medications could be produced from dates. Dates are able to eliminate germs and worms, they help solve hearing problems, they protect vascular walls, they do not raise cholesterol, they help generate urine, they help prevent stones in the bladder, and they alkalize the blood, for they are rich in alkalizing salts that decrease the probability of kidney and gallbladder disease, as well as gout. Dates also enhance the reproductive system with their phosphorus, zinc and other vital minerals and nutrients.

Efficiency during School Examinations

As previously explained, dates are a nerve tranquillizer that cast away anger and calm hyperactive and uneasy children. Therefore, they are quite suitable for children taking examinations, which can be a very stressful time.

Dates have an above-average nutritional value. Among fruits, they are also the least affected by decay and contamination. Dates and their seeds have numerous benefits in addition to those we have already described, both industrial and economical.

The numerous advantages of dates can be broadly described and science is still discovering them. Dates are the food of Maryam (⌘) and they are the food of the fasting Muslim, as well.

Dates: Food for Those Who Fast and a Remedy for Patients

Despite the inexpensive price and availability of dates in stores, many scientists name them "the manjam," which means, "the gold mine." Why? Because dates are rich in many essential elements and they are beneficial for the human body. Dates are mentioned repeatedly in the Qur'ān and in sūratu-l-maryam, verses 25-26 (see page 20).

One kilogram of dates has the same nutritional value as meat! What is their secret?

Dates include a relatively higher percentage of vitamin A than foods considered to be this vitamin's source, such as fish oil and butter. This vitamin helps infants grow and enhances vision, especially at night.

Bananas in the Holy Qur'an

Bananas reduce gastric acidity and help heal lung diseases and kidney ulcers. They increase urine generation, sperm generation and sexual desire, and they soften the stomach. However, bananas are fattening and consuming large amounts of them may cause stomach problems, jaundice or excess phlegm, which can be treated with cane sugar, honey and ginger. Therefore, bananas should be eaten before meals.

The greatest nutritional value is found in the ripest, sweetest and largest bananas. Cooking them in almond oil or sesame oil and then applying that oil to the scalp can help an itchy scalp. Also, cooking bananas with watermelon seeds and then applying this oil to the face removes freckles, softens the skin, improves skin color and prevents swellings.

Bananas are beneficial for coughs, chest pain, rough tracheas, lean kidneys and ischemia.[15]

Using vinegar or lemon juice as an ointment can treat baldness or hair loss, chronic inflammation of the eyelids, itchiness and allergies.

Watermelon juice helps get rid of freckles, softens the skin and improves its color. The ashes of burnt watermelon peel help wounds to heal and stops bleeding. Place watermelon leaves on swellings to heal them.

---

[15] Restriction in blood supply generally due to factors in the blood vessels that create tissue damage or dysfunction.

Banana's Medicinal Uses

1. Hypertension
Bananas, with their high levels of potassium and low levels of sodium, as well as their cholesterol-free nutrition, help cure hypertension. Therefore, bananas are a hypertension patient's favorite food!

2. Gastric Acidity and Diarrhea
Bananas contain high levels of potassium, which is an alkalizing salt that moderates stomach acidity. Potassium that is easily digested can be used to treat stomach ulcers.

3. Gastrointestinal Disorders
It is advised to consume bananas frequently, for they improve the functioning of both the digestive system and the intestines.

4. Malnutrition and Vitamin Deficiency
Bananas contain relatively high levels of vitamins A, B-complex and C, as well as providing carbohydrates. Therefore, they are recommended for malnutrition.

5. Pellagra
Bananas are rich in niacin, a vitamin that protects people from pellagra. This disease is most common in poor countries whose foods have very limited nutritional value.

Pellagra's symptoms include: cracked and dry skin; dark spots on the hands, face, neck and feet; rough skin; burning skin that drives patients to scratch these irritating areas, which results in blisters and infections; inflammation of the mucous membranes; tongue inflammation, which is followed by loss of appetite, vomiting and diarrhea; migraines; numbness in the limbs; damage to the spinal cord; hallucinations; irritability and insanity.

Please note that even though niacin is easily digested and absorbed into our bodies, it is not affected by high temperatures, light, alkalizing or oxidizing agents. Therefore, it can be stored and preserved for a long time.

6. Childhood Development and Growth
Children require very rich nutrition during their initial stages of growth. Therefore, in order to help them grow and develop healthy bodies, they need to eat bananas. Bananas also provide psychological balance and pleasant feelings.

7. Recommended for…
Bananas are recommended for convalescents, the elderly, anemic patients, people suffering from continuous weakness, and people suffering from kidneys leaking protein into the urine (microalbuminuria).

8. Bananas Are Nutrition and Strengthen the Muscles
Generally, they are boosting and a certain cure for leanness. They activate the kidneys and the urinary system in the elderly.

9. Bananas Balance Overall Health
Bananas help us to develop intelligence and they stimulate brain and memory function. Therefore, bananas were named by our ancestors, "food of the philosophers."

Bananas also:

- Protect teeth from decay and cavities.
- Efficiently regulate the nervous system.
- Prevent diseases of the colon (i.e. diverticulitis) and give the body abundant energy.
- Benefit the proper functioning of the reproductive organs and they benefit both pregnant and breastfeeding women.

- Protect the body from lung diseases, as well as kidney and bladder ulcers; they also help generate urine.
- Are useful for gas and indigestion when eaten baked with flour.
- Increase sperm production and the desire for sexual intercourse.
- Soften the stomach.
- Heal peptic ulcer disease.
- Decrease the level of cholesterol in the body (immature banana fibers are used to treat this disease).
- Nourish and soften the body.
- Heal scurvy.
- Energize the body.
- Provide very efficient nutrition for workers, the elderly and pregnant women.
- Prevent sclerosis[16] and arteriosclerosis.
- Contribute to better thinking and meditation.
- Cure diarrhea.
- Decrease hypertension.
- Do not cause obesity.
- Treat malnutrition when eaten with coconuts.
- Cure obesity and kidney diseases.
- Banana root extract treats jaundice, headaches and measles.
- Banana juice serves as a snake bite remedy.

---

[16] Stiffening of the kidneys.

Bananas Treat Obesity and Kidney Disease

It is said that the name "banana" was taken from the Arabs, for they named it after the word "banan" which means "fingers" in Arabic (which this fruit resembles). Bananas are found in Spain and Morocco and they are in the top tier of rich, nutritious foods for the human body. A meal consisting of banana, milk and bread provides the body with everything it needs.

In addition, bananas help treat sponge-like obesity[17] and edema or hydropsy.[18] The healing process occurs because bananas provide the body with heat and extra energy and they moderate the level of salts in the body. The potassium in this fruit adds to its numerous medical and nutritional benefits because potassium relieves the pressure of the kidneys and arteries. Therefore, it is an essential and vital food for those with a kidney disease.

However, bananas are not preferred as a stand-alone meal, for they alone cannot achieve the body's optimal nutritional balance. If bananas are frequently eaten as meals, it might cause digestive disorders and anemia. Bananas are rich in minerals and vitamins, especially vitamin C, which is beneficial for treating scurvy, exhaustion and fatigue, rheumatism, inflammation of the nerves and inactive intelligence.

Patients suffering from chronic constipation should not consume high amounts of banana, for it is low in dietary fiber, which is necessary for helping the body dispose of waste. This is also true for diabetic patients, for bananas contain of a high proportion of starch.

Bananas should be chewed properly and not swallowed immediately. It is not recommended to eat artificially-ripened bananas, which have lost much of their nutritional value and benefit.

---

[17] A result of excessive fluid storage.
[18] An abnormal accumulation of fluid beneath the skin.

Bananas in the Diet

Bananas are usually picked when they are still unripe. It is preferable to buy bananas when they are half-ripe and to let them sit until they ripen. Ripe bananas are either dark yellow or bright yellow, according to type. Unripe bananas can also be eaten for certain purposes and they can be cooked with other types of fruit. From very ripe dried bananas you can make banana flour, just as flour is made from dried vegetables.

Banana flour is similar to rice flour in its chemical structure. In France, there is a kind of bread made from banana flour specifically for patients who suffer from excess protein in the urine. In other countries, people eat this kind of bread grilled or with butter. In India and Sudan, banana flour is kneaded with sugar, baked and then perfumed and used as travel food.

The Medicinal Use of Garlic

Garlic is considered an antibiotic, as well as a cure for many diseases. Garlic is used in the treatment of the following diseases:

How to Do a Garlic Steam

Garlic steams are recommended in many of the remedies below.

1. Chop a handful of garlic and add it to a saucepan, along with some water.

2. Bring the garlic water to a boil and then lower the heat, keeping it at a soft simmer.

3. Inhale the steam for several minutes.

1. Poisoning / Toxicity

1. Mash 5 cloves of garlic.

2. Boil some black seed in water and sweeten it with ¼ cup of honey.

3. Then, mix the mashed garlic with the honey and black seed mixture. Drink it immediately, in the morning and at night and you will heal, inshā'a-llāh (ﷻ).

2. Stomach Cleansing

1. Swallow 1 clove of chopped garlic on an empty stomach.

2. Immediately afterward, drink 1 cup of boiled cumin sweetened with honey.

3. Repeat this daily for a week.

3. Dissolve Cholesterol and Prevent Blood Clots

1. At lunchtime, add 2 mashed cloves of garlic to a bowl of salad. Eat this salad daily.

- Garlic has been proven to be an effective treatment for hypertension. However, do not continue to eat garlic once your blood pressure has reached its normal level, otherwise, it will continue to lower. People with low blood pressure should reduce their garlic intake.

4. Increase Urination and Cleanse the Urinary Tract

1. Boil some barley well, strain the water and allow it to cool.

2. Mash 3 cloves of garlic and add it to the cooled barley water.

3. Drink this mixture every day on an empty stomach.

4. In addition, drink as much lemon juice as possible, as well as other soft drinks (not soda).

5. Amoeba and Dysentery

- Eat 1 chopped clove of garlic after every meal for a week, following it with 1 teaspoon of olive oil.

6. Dyspepsia, Stomach Gas and Abdominal Cramps

1. Add 3 cloves of garlic to 1 cup of pear juice.

2. Drink before bedtime every day or when there is pain.

3. In addition, massage the stomach with garlic oil and olive oil.

7. Typhoid

1. Chop 5 cloves of garlic and mix them with 1 cup of hot milk sweetened with honey. Drink before bedtime.

2. Apply some garlic and olive oil to the patient's spinal cord and limbs. In the morning, the patient should do a garlic steam for 5 minutes.

8. Chronic Ulcers

1. Mash some garlic cloves until they are smooth.

2. Apply them as an ointment to the ulcer and then bandage the wound.

•   You can cleanse the wound with a mixture of mashed garlic and warm water, which eradicates the microbes in the wound.

9. Diphtheria

1. Chew 1 clove of garlic for 3 minutes. Then swallow it. Repeat after every meal, daily.

2. Afterward, do a garlic steam for 5 minutes.

3. These steps should be done for 3 days, being cautious not to catch a cold while doing so.

10. To Strengthen and Calm the Nervous System

1. Chop 1 clove of garlic and add it to 1 cup of hot milk along with several drops of amber oil.

2. Drink this mixture on an empty stomach, for it enhances and calms the nervous system.

11. Deafness from Accident or Infection

1. Press 7 cloves of garlic and cook them on low heat in olive oil.

2. As it cools, put several drops of the oil into the ears before bedtime and seal each ear with cotton.

3. Repeat every day for as long as it is useful.

12. The Flu

1. Press 7 cloves of garlic and mix them with orange juice and lemon juice.

2. Drink on an empty stomach every day.

3. In addition, do a garlic steam before bedtime.

4. After this regime is repeated once or twice, the flu will be gone, inshā'a-llāh (﷾).

13. Common Cold

1. Swallow 1 clove of garlic and drink a mixture of lemon juice and pressed garlic after every meal.

2. Also, do a garlic steam, for it is very helpful in healing colds.

14. Cancer

- Garlic contains a substance called alpine, which is known to be part of garlic's anti-cancer properties. Therefore, every patient should consistently eat a lot of garlic and carrots.

15. Whooping Cough

1. Before going to sleep, do a garlic steam. Add a pinch of salt to the garlic water before bringing it to a boil.

2. Keep the garlic water warm until the next morning and then do another steam. This is repeated each morning and night for a week.

16. Tuberculosis

1. Every morning, mash 3 cloves of garlic and spread them on a piece of bread. Eat the garlic bread on an empty stomach.

2. In the evening, do a garlic steam.

3. This should be repeated for 1 month.

17. Cholera

- In order to be protected from cholera while it is spreading, have 1 teaspoon of garlic paste and honey after every meal.

18. Parasites and Worms

1. Mash 3 cloves of garlic and mix them with 1 cup of milk without sugar.

2. Drink this mixture morning and night before bedtime.

3. Have a drink of castor oil and repeat this now and then to completely cleanse the stomach of parasites.

19. Scabies

1. Chop 5 cloves of garlic and mix them with butter.

2. Apply this mixture to the affected areas morning and night and take a bath in the morning.

3. Continue doing so for a week. This will totally cleanse the skin.

20. Gallstones

1. Mix ½ cup of mashed garlic with 1 cup of lemon juice, 1 cup of olive oil, and a handful of fresh, chopped parsley.

2. Take 1 teaspoon of this mixture daily with plenty of water.

21. Dandruff

1. Press 3 whole heads of garlic until they become paste.

2. Mix the garlic with apple cider vinegar and let it sit in a flask in sunny a place for 1 week.

3. Massage the scalp with the paste daily for a week. This remedy will eradicate dandruff, in addition to softening the hair.

4. After 1 week of using this remedy, apply some olive oil several times to the scalp.

22. To Strengthen Memory and as a General Tonic

1. Blend 3 cloves of garlic, 3 tomatoes and a little salt in a blender.

2. Drink this as a cold juice at any time, for it is a stimulant for both the body and mind.

23. To Strengthen the Gums and Prevent Tooth Loss

1. Mash some cloves of garlic and massage your gums with your index finger.

2. Gargle with a mixture of parsley boiled in water. Have some mint to remove the garlic odor.

24. To Enhance Sexual Ability

1. Mash some garlic and cook on low heat with olive oil until it becomes yellowish. Put it in a small flask to preserve it.

2. Apply it, when needed, to the root of the urethra (pubis) by massaging it in a circular motion. This should not be washed for at least 1 hour.

25. Headaches

1. Apply some garlic oil to the head (the area that aches) and it will be as if you never had the headache.

2. To enhance this remedy, chop a clove of garlic and swallow it with some water.

26. Dizziness

- Have an omelet made from eggs, garlic and olive oil 3 times a day for 3 days in a row. This will totally vanquish dizziness. You can add salt and spices in the omelet, as well.

27. Tooth Pain

1. Put ½ clove of garlic where it hurts. Wait a while and soon the pain will end.

2. If the tooth pain overwhelms a larger part of the jaw, then put 1 clove of garlic in the inner section of the outer ear (pinna), parallel to the side of the hurting jaw.

28. Muscle Building and Strength

1. Drink a large glass of milk with 1 or 2 chopped cloves of garlic on an empty stomach. Repeat every day for 1 month.

2. Then, do not do this at all for 1 month.

3. After the month-long break is over, begin the routine again. This helps in building a stronger body, no matter what your age.

29. Hypertension and Arteriosclerosis

1. Press some garlic and heat it in olive oil.

2. Preserve it in a jar away from the sun for 40 days.

3. Take 1 teaspoon of it on an empty stomach for 40 days.

30. Protection from Plague and AIDS

1. Drink garlic juice by adding 3 cloves of garlic to 1 cup of honey and water on a daily basis.

2. This will be the cure, inshā'a-llāh (﷾).

31. Eye Diseases and Problems

- Chew garlic leaves and put them on the infected eye morning and night, for they even heal ophthalmia and trachoma (severe eye diseases).

32. Hypertension

- It is enough to consistently swallow 1 clove of garlic daily to heal this disease.

  Note: Garlic reduces hypertension because it reduces the cholesterol and fat levels in the blood. In addition, it activates the heart's work and boosts circulation.

The Medicinal Use of Onion

Onions are one of the most ancient vegetables and they are highly valued for their nutrition. They were used in facial massage to add a youthful look to the skin. Its seeds are known to eradicate skin pigmentation, in addition to having numerous benefits for different diseases.

How to Prepare an Onion Poultice

Preparing an onion poultice is important for the treatment of many diseases, as you will read below. To do so:

1. Slice or chop several onions and then heat them.

2. Cover the infected area(s) with the onions and cover the onions with a piece of cloth that is thicker than wool in order to preserve the heat.

3. Tie the cloth around the affected body part in order to keep the onions in place. Change this poultice every 12 hours.

1. Whooping Cough

1. Cook some onions in water with some sugar cane until the liquids become as thick as honey. Preserve the liquid in a jar and have 1 teaspoon of it after every meal, daily.

2. Have children take 1 teaspoon 3 times a day.

2. Asthma

1. Mix onion juice and honey.

2. Take ¼ cup of this mixture morning and night for 1 month. This is very beneficial for asthma, inshā'a-llāh (﷽).

3. Pneumonia

- Put an onion poultice on the chest and cover it with a cloth before bedtime. This helps eliminate pneumonia, inshā'a-llāh (﷽).

4. Prostate Disease

1. Soak some onions in apple cider vinegar for 3 days.

2. Drink ¼ cup on an empty stomach for 10 days in a row.

5. Painful or Difficult Urination

1. Chop onions into rings and heat.

2. Place them in a poultice over the right and left kidneys and on the area above the bladder and under the navel.

3. Also, drink a mixture of onion juice, lemon juice, honey and hot water once or twice.

6. To Provide Strength and Activity

- Drink a mixture of onion juice, tomato juice and a little salt, for this energizes the human body at any time.

Another remedy:

1. Cook mutton with onions and then put it in the blender with 1 cup of wheat juice.

2. Drink this mixture like a soup 2 hours after lunch. It provides the body with vitality and strength.

Or:

1. One can also grind radish seeds and mix them with onion juice.

2. Eat olive oil, cheese and finely ground thyme. This is a powerful energizer.

7. Reproductive Enhancement

1. Place 1 cup of honey and ½ cup onion in a saucepan and bring to a boil.

2. Cook until the onion odor totally disappears.

3. Take 1 teaspoon of this mixture after every meal.

4. It is also advised to have grilled onions with peanuts, dates and honey, which is also a wondrous remedy.

8. Psychological Diseases

- Boil unpeeled onions and then eat them.

Or:

- Drink a blend of onion juice, lettuce and 1 teaspoon of honey. This should be drunk while cold.

9. Rheumatism

1. Chop a large onion and cook it in water until it begins to produce a lot of steam.

2. Apply some olive oil to the affected joint and then steam the joint with the onion water for several minutes (put the pot under the body part and allow the steam to warm the area for several minutes). While doing this, massage the rheumatic area.

3. In the morning, have 1 teaspoon of thyme mixed with about ¼ cup of honey.

4. Do this for 1 week.

10. Bruising

1. Combine equal amounts of onion juice and eucalyptus oil and massage the bruise morning and evening.

2. While using this treatment, try not to move or strain the injured area.

11. Broken Bones and the Pain Associated with Them

1. Prepare onion soup with bone marrow (preferably camel bones, but if they are unavailable cow bones will do). You may spice this soup as desired.

2. Drink the soup daily for lunch.

3. After removing the splint from the fractured area, eat lots of onions, for they will accelerate the healing process and enhance the nerves.

12. Cancerous Sores

1. Mix ¼ cup onion juice with about 1 teaspoon of stinging nettle juice.

2. Apply this combination to the cancerous sores every day.

3. In addition, drink 1 teaspoon of the same mixture and follow it with 1 cup of milk sweetened with honey.

13. Abscesses

1. Chop an onion and heat it with olive oil over low heat.

2. Remove the onion from the heat before it begin to get yellow, apply it as an ointment to the infected area, and cover it with a bandage.

3. Clean the area and change the bandage every day until the pus fully expresses and then is gone.

4. Then apply black seed oil to the affected area.

14. Septic Wounds

1. Mix together some chopped onions and olive oil or honey.

2. Smear the mixture onto the wound every day, for it is a cure inshāʾa-llāh (ﷻ).

15. Varicose Veins

1. Prepare a poultice containing husked onions and the same amount of chopped comfrey.

2. Bandage the treated area and leave the poultice on from evening to morning.

3. Repeat this treatment daily for 1 week.

16. Chilblains in Winter

1. Prepare a poultice with heated onions and place it on the area to treat (hand, feet, etc.) in the evening before bedtime. Leave the poultice on until the morning.

2. Remove it, wash the area and then massage some olive oil into the infected area.

17. Headaches

1. Boil husked onions with ground cloves.

2. Mix with olive oil and leave to cool.

3. Strain the mixture, saving the liquid. Use the liquid to massage the area on the head that hurts.

4. In addition, eat 1 teaspoon of the mixture before bedtime. Inshā'a-llāh (ﷻ), this treatment will heal the nervous system.

18. Acne

1. Boil an onion and mash it up.

2. Mix it with wheat flour, 1 egg and 1 teaspoon of sesame oil.

3. Apply the paste to the infected areas morning and evening.

4. Eat plenty of onions to cleanse the stomach and bloodstream.

19. Eczema

1. Clean the affected areas with some diluted vinegar.

2. Prepare a paste of onion juice and wild thyme and smear it on the infected areas.

3. Repeat daily. Also, eat plenty of fresh fruits and vegetables, as well as bread and honey.

20. Skin Cancer

1. Blend together the juice of 1 onion, some ground fenugreek seed and ¼ teaspoon of yellow sulfate.

2. Prepare the ointment and apply it to the infected area daily.

3. In the evening, wash the area and then apply olive oil to it.

4. This treatment should be repeated for a week.

21. Kidney Diseases and Kidney Stones

1. Take an unpeeled onion and stuff it with roasted, ground date pits.

2. Cook the stuffed onion.

3. Eat this every day for a week and it will heal the kidney from inflammation, stones and salts.

22. Ascites

1. Prepare onion soup by boiling 3 onions for 15 minutes in water.

2. Strain the broth and drink it after every meal.

23. Coughing (for Children and Adults)

1. Chop an onion and leave it in 1 cup of honey for 3 hours.

2. Eat 1 teaspoon of the honey after every meal.

3. This remedy helps purify the blood and body from salts. Make eating onions a habit, especially with cheese and olive oil, for that combination is definitely a detergent for the body and the blood.

24. Diabetes

1. Eat an onion every day, for onions reduce blood sugar levels.

2. Then eat cabbage seeds, for they eradicate diabetes and stop frequent urination.

25. Diphtheria

1. Dry sauté some onions (with no oil or butter) over low heat.

2. Put the onions in a poultice and place it on the throat and beneath the lower jaw every day, covering it with a bandage or gauze.

3. Drink a mixture of onion juice and warm water every morning and evening.

26. Tonsillitis

1. Place a poultice of heated onion around the neck and on the throat.

2. Gargle with onion juice and honey 3 times a day.

27. Ear Diseases

1. Place a poultice of heated onions behind the auricle of the ear.

2. Mix some onion juice and olive oil and drink some of it in the morning and at night. Clean the ear between treatments.

28. Spleen

1. Stuff some unpeeled onions with a mixture of black seed and fennel.

2. Grill the onions and then eat the onion like a sandwich with some olive oil, cheese and grilled spleen.

3. This meal is very beneficial for the spleen. This meal can be prepared every 2 or 3 days.

29. Hair Loss

1. Massage onion juice into the scalp before bedtime.

2. Wash it in the morning with warm water until your hair stops falling out.

30. Dizziness

1. Remove the onion root from an unpeeled onion with the intention of creating a space within it to stuff coriander.

2. Stuff the onion with coriander and replace the root to close up the onion.

3. Grill the onion and eat it like a sandwich with cheese or butter.

31. Eye Diseases and Cataracts

1. Combine equal amounts of onion juice and honey.

2. Drop several drops of this mixture into the infected eye, for this is the best remedy.

32. Weight Loss

These remedies help you to enjoy a healthy and athletic body, as well as melt body fat, lose your potbelly and solidify areas of flabbiness. These tips can be used by men and women. Do as follows:

- Drink 1 teaspoon of onion juice daily. It can be mixed with fruit juice.

- Drink an emulsion of alchemilla (Lady's Mantle) morning and evening.

- Maintain late night prayers and meditate while reciting the Qur'ān. Beware of having more for dinner than 1 cup of yogurt with some fruit.

- Exercise daily (jogging and so on).

33. Common Cold

1. Place a poultice of heated onions on the neck, close to the hair.

2. In addition, do an onion steam (boil chopped onions over low heat and inhale the onion steam).

34. The Flu

1. Eat 1 onion before going to sleep at night.

2. Immediately drink the juice of 1 lemon and some of its peel.

35. Coughing

1. Boil equal amounts of onion juice and honey.

2. Drink 1 teaspoon of the mixture after every meal.

3. Place an onion poultice on the chest and cover it with paper or gauze before sleeping.

36. Hypotension

1. Mix 1 teaspoon of onion juice and 1 teaspoon of Genista tinctoria (dyer's broom) in a cup of hot water until the mixture is emulsified.

2. Drink like a tea in the evening before going to sleep.

37. Angina Pectoris

1. Massage the chest with onion oil.

2. Drink 1 cup of an emulsion of the Achilles plant. To prepare an emulsion of this plant, soak it in cold water for 5 minutes.

3. Strain it and drink 1 cup of the thick liquid on an empty stomach.

38. Indigestion

1. Boil an onion with its peel. After it is soft, peel it and mash it with honey.

2. Make a sandwich with the mixture and eat it. It is enhanced when eaten with dates, fennel, black seed, thyme and cheese.

39. Worms and Parasites

- Inject the patient with an enema filled with boiled onion. This will eliminate the parasites and worms.

40. For Youthfulness, Energy and Strength

1. Grill some onions with their peels.

2. When ready, remove the peels and mash the onions with honey and butter.

3. Eat this mixture with wheat bread as a sandwich for breakfast. Then drink ½ liter of milk.

41. Mouth Cleanser

- It has been proven that chewing onion for few minutes is quite enough to cleanse the mouth from all infectious microbes, such as diphtheria microbes.

42. Wound Sterilizer

- Using an onion steam is an effective way to sterilize wounds and help them to heal, inshā'a-llāh (ﷻ). To prepare an onion steam, follow the directions in the rheumatism remedy on page 59.

43. To Prevent Thrombosis

- Onions prevent the formation of blood clots. Onions are considered the most important preventative remedy for heart health. For patients who suffer from vulnerable hearts: persistently eat onions as a main element in your diet to help prevent angina pectoris and other heart traumas.

The Medicinal Use of Black Seed (Nigella sativa)

Black seed (the seed of blessing) has abundant benefits for healing and treating disease. The Prophet Muḥammad (ﷺ) said:

> There is healing in black seed for all diseases except death.
> (Bukhārī 71:592)

Black seed oil is the preferred form of black seed for treating disease. This oil is extracted only after the seeds are ripe and dried. When the seeds turn black, they are ready. As you are about to learn from the following remedies, when black seed is mentioned it usually refers to black seed oil.

1. Hair Loss
1. Mix ground black seed with some arugula juice, 1 teaspoon of diluted vinegar and ¼ cup of olive oil.

2. Massage the head with this mixture every evening.

3. Wash with warm water and soap in the morning.

2. Headaches
1. Mix the following: 2 parts ground black seed, 1 part finely ground cloves, 1 part anise and some black seed oil.

2. Take as much as you desire when you have a headache, in addition to black seed oil.

3. Sleeping Disorders
- Mix 1 teaspoon of black seed oil in a cup of hot milk sweetened with honey and drink it.

4. Dizziness and Earache
1. Put 1 drop of black seed oil into the aching ear to cleanse it.

2. Drink some black seed oil, as well.

3. Dizziness is healed by massaging the temples and the back of the head with black seed oil.

5. Alopecia from Infection

1. Mix together 1 teaspoon of finely ground black seed, ¼ cup of diluted apple cider vinegar and 1 teaspoon of garlic juice. You are going to use this mixture like an ointment and apply it to the infected area after shaving it.

2. Apply the mixture to the infected area and then bandage it. Leave it on your head from morning until night.

3. Smear some black seed oil on the area after removing the bandage. This should be repeated daily for a week.

6. Herpes

- Apply some black seed oil to the herpes sores and after several days they will be gone, inshā'a-llāh (ﷻ).

7. Gynecological Diseases and Labor

- One of the most effective facilitators of labor is black seed oil sweetened with honey and added to chamomile tea.

- Black seed is also a wonderful topical remedy for women during and after labor.

- Using a few drops of black seed oil in every drink will both immunize women from and cure all gynecological diseases.

8. To Protect the Teeth and Treat the Throat

1. Boil some black seed and as it cools, gargle with it to cleanse the mouth and throat from disease.

2. Take 1 teaspoon of black seed oil on an empty stomach and follow it with warm water. This should be repeated daily.

3. In addition, massage the throat and gums with black seed oil.

9. Endocrine Diseases and Disorders
1. Mix some finely ground black seed with honey and royal jelly.

2. Eat some of this mixture daily for a month.

10. Acne
1. Add ground black seed to sesame oil and mix well with 1 teaspoon of wheat flour.

2. Apply the paste to the face and the infected areas in the evening. In the morning, wash with warm water and soap.

3. This should be repeated for a week. To enhance the remedy, add black seed oil to any beverage or drink.

11. Skin Disorders
1. Mix 1 part black seed oil and 1 part flower oil with 2 parts whole wheat flour.

2. Sterilize the infected area by wiping it with a cloth dampened in diluted vinegar. Then expose the area to the sun.

3. Every day apply some of the mixture to the infected area.

4. Avoid allergy-causing foods like fish, eggs and mango.

12. Vitiligo and Leprosy
1. Mix together 1 teaspoon of black seed, vinegar, henna and ground dried chameleon leather. Add vinegar, if necessary, to soften the dough.

2. Apply this paste to the infected skin and leave it on from morning until night.

3. This is repeated daily and the treated areas should be exposed to the sun.

13. Facial Cosmetic
1. Mix finely ground black seed with olive oil and then apply it to the face.

2. Expose your face to sun (but not excessively).

14. Help Broken Bones Heal More Quickly

1. Apply this treatment after removing the splint from the affected area.

2. Mix together some honey, onion, boiled egg and 1 teaspoon of finely ground black seed.

3. Apply this mixture to the treated area daily while massaging it.

4. Also, massage the areas adjacent to the broken bone with warm black seed oil.

15. Bruising and Fractures

1. Boil a handful of black seed in a pot full of water and then allow it to cool somewhat.

2. Dip the fractured limb in the water or simply pour the liquid on the affected area and let it soak for 15 minutes or more.

3. While doing so, try to carefully move the limb.

4. Afterward, apply black seed oil on the fractured area before bedtime.

5. Do not strain or stress the affected limb.

16. Rheumatism

1. Heat black seed oil and massage the rheumatic area with it strongly, as if you were massaging the bones and not the skin.

2. Also, drink heated black seed sweetened with honey before bedtime.

17. Diabetes

1. Grind 1 cup of black seed into a fine powder.

2. Mix the black seed powder with 1 teaspoon of finely ground Commiphora molmol,[19] ½ cup of garden cress seeds,[20] 1 cup of freeze-dried pomegranate powder, 1 cup of ground dried cabbage root and 1 teaspoon of asafetida (Ferula asafoetida).

3. Every day, eat 1 teaspoon of this mixture with yogurt on an empty stomach.

18. Hypertension

1. Add a few drops of black seed oil to every hot beverage.

2. This remedy has an even greater effect when you apply black seed oil to your whole body and sunbathe once a week.

19. Kidney Infections

1. Prepare a poultice of black seed powder and olive oil.

2. Place the poultice on the side of the painful kidney.

3. Take 1 teaspoon of black seed oil on an empty stomach every day for 1 week.

4. The infection will be healed, inshā'a-llāh (ﷻ).

20. To Dissolve and Eliminate Kidney Stones

1. Grind ¼ cup of black seed and mix it with 1 cup of honey.

2. Chop 3 cloves of garlic and add it to the mixture.

3. Take ⅓ of the mixture 3 times a day.

4. Repeat this treatment for several days, in addition to eating 1 whole lemon with its peel each time (afterward). This will cleanse and sterilize the kidneys.

---

[19] Commiphora is a genus of flowering plants that includes about 185 species of trees and shrubs, often armed or thorny, native to Africa, Arabia and the Indian subcontinent. Included are myrrh and Balsam of Mecca.

[20] Garden cress (Lapidium sativum) is related to watercress and mustard, sharing their peppery, tangy flavor and aroma. In some regions, garden cress is known as garden pepper cress, pepper grass, pepperwort or poor man's pepper.

21. Difficult or Painful Urination

1. Massage the pubic area with black seed oil before bedtime.

2. Also, drink 1 cup of boiled black seed in water sweetened with honey afterward.

3. Do this every day until the problem is healed.

22. Preventing Involuntary Urination

1. Wash and clean some eggshells properly.

2. Roast and grind them; then add some black seed oil.

3. Drink 1 teaspoon of the mixture with 1 cup of yogurt daily, for 1 week.

4. This can be drunk at any time during the day.

23. Dropsy

1. Prepare a poultice containing a paste comprised of ground black seed and vinegar.

2. Put a piece of gauze on the navel. Then put the paste on the navel.

3. Drink 1 teaspoon of black seed oil in the morning and evening for a week.

4. Inshā'a-llāh (﷾), this remedy will reveal His mighty, tremendous ability to heal these diseases.

24. Hepatitis (Liver Infections)

This remedy requires lots of patience and after patience comes relief, inshā'a-llāh (﷾).

1. Add 1 teaspoon of ground black seed to ¼ teaspoon of prickly pear fruit and mix it with honey.

2. Eat some of this mixture on an empty stomach every day for 2 consecutive months.

25. Meningitis

1. Boil a mixture of dried sea urchin skin and black seed.

2. Inhale the steam from the boiling mixture for several minutes.

3. Drink black seed oil with lemon juice morning and night.

- Inshā'a-llāh ta'ālā (ﷺ), beginning from the first day treated, the patient will no longer have a fever.

26. Gallbladder Diseases and Stones

1. Add 1 teaspoon of black seed to ¼ teaspoon of Commiphora molmol and mix them with 1 cup of honey. Prepare and eat this entire mixture in the morning and then again at night.

2. This should be repeated daily until the face gets red, which means that the gallbladder has been healed inshā'a-llāh (ﷺ). So thank Him (ﷺ) for His innumerable blessings and grace.

27. Spleen Diseases

1. Prepare a poultice comprised of a mixture of black seed and olive oil heated on low for a few minutes.

2. Place the poultice on the left side beneath the left ribs at night.

3. At the same time, drink some boiled fenugreek tea sweetened with honey, with several drops of black seed oil added.

4. After 2 weeks of continuous treatment, the patient will see inshā'a-llāh (ﷺ), that the spleen is healed. Thank Him for that.

28. Lung Diseases and Cold

1. Before bedtime, cook 1 teaspoon of black seed oil in some water until it begins to steam. Inhale the steam.

2. In addition, drink 1 cup of boiled thyme and black seed powder every day, morning and night until the illness is totally over.

29. The Heart and the Circulatory System

Be confident in our Prophet Muḥammad's sayings (ﷺ),
for this is one of the requirements of imān (faith).
When the Prophet (ﷺ) tells us that black seed cures
every disease humanity is tested with,
then surely it is unquestionably
the cure for all diseases.

- A person suffering from heart disease should not despair of Allāh's mercy (ﷻ). He should simply consume a lot of black seed with honey at any time of the day and he will be healed.

30. Intestinal Colic

1. Boil equal amounts of anise, cumin and peppermint leaves in water.

2. Sweeten the mixture with a little bit of sugar cane or honey.

3. Add 7 drops of black seed oil while it is still hot.

4. Drink it and apply some black seed oil to the area that hurts. In minutes the pain will be over, inshā'a-llāh (ﷻ).

31. Diarrhea

1. Mix 1 teaspoon of finely ground black seed with arugula juice.

2. Drink 1 cup of this mixture 3 times a day until the diarrhea stops (normally the second day).

3. Stop the treatment the moment the diarrhea stops so as not to have constipation.

32. Nausea

1. Boil some carnation with black seed and drink it with no added sweeteners 3 times a day until the nausea stops.

33. Gas and Cramps

1. Take 1 teaspoon of finely ground black seed and follow it with 1 cup of hot water sweetened with 3 teaspoons of honey.

2. This should be repeated daily for a week.

34. Acid Reflux

1. Mix several drops of black seed oil and some honey or sugar cane in a cup of hot yogurt.

2. Inshā'a-llāh (﷾) the acidity will end as if it had never existed.

35. Colon Pain and Reactivation

1. Mix 1 teaspoon of finely ground black seed and 1 teaspoon of licorice root (Glycyrrhiza glabra) in a cup of pear juice.

2. Drink it and behold its wondrous ability to eliminate colon pain while reactivating it. It is also a known way remedy for totally relaxing the nervous system, inshā'a-llāh (﷾).

36. Eye Diseases

1. Massage both temples, the areas closer to the eyes, and the eyelids with black seed oil before bedtime.

2. Add several drops of black seed oil to any hot beverage (or carrot juice).

37. Amoebiasis

1. Mix finely ground black seed with 1 teaspoon of mashed garlic in a cup of salted, hot tomato sauce.

2. Drink it on an empty stomach daily for 2 continuous weeks. The infection will be over inshā'a-llāh (﷾).

38. Schistosomiasis (snail fever)

1. Take 1 teaspoon of finely ground black seed morning and evening (you can eat it with bread and cheese).

2. Apply black seed oil to the right side of your body before bedtime.

3. Continue doing so for 3 months.

39. Parasites and Worms

1. Mix 1 teaspoon of finely ground black seed, 3 chopped cloves of garlic, 1 teaspoon of olive oil, some spices and 10 gourd seeds.

2. Make it into a sandwich and eat it in the morning, followed by a drink of fennel or castor oil (once).

40. Infertility

1. The following 3 things are always available thanks to Allāh ta'ālā (☀). Mix equal amounts of black seed powder, finely ground fenugreek and radish seeds together.

2. Combine 1 teaspoon of this mixture with ½ cup of honey and eat it in the morning and evening.

3. Follow it with a big cup of camel's milk.[21]

4. Inshā'a-llāh (☀), your desire will be fulfilled.

41. Prostate Health

1. Massage the lower part of the back with black seed oil and then massage the bottom of the testicles using circular motions.

2. Drink a mixture of 1 teaspoon of finely ground black seed and ¼ teaspoon of myrrh in ½ cup of honey, diluted with some warm water.

3. This should be done at any time of day on a daily basis.

---

[21] You cannot substitute a different type of milk. If you cannot acquire camel's milk in the U.S., have it shipped from elsewhere.

42. Asthma

1. Cook some black seed in water until it begins to steam.

2. Inhale the black seed steam in the morning and in the evening.

3. Also, eat 1 teaspoon of black seed powder in the morning before breakfast and in the evening.

4. In addition, apply black seed oil to the chest and throat before bedtime daily.

43. Gastric Ulcers

1. Combine 10 drops of black seed oil with ¼ cup of honey and 1 teaspoon of finely ground pomegranate and eat this mixture when your stomach is empty. Follow it by eating 1 cup of unsweetened yogurt.

2. By Allāh's blessing (﷾), when this mixture is taken persistently every day for 2 months, the ulcers will be completely healed.

44. Cancer

1. Rub the body with black seed oil 3 times a day.

2. Take 1 teaspoon of black seed powder after every meal with a cup of carrot juice.

3. Continue to apply this treatment regularly for 3 months.

4. In addition, do not stop your prayers and reciting the Qur'ān.

5. Soon the patient will notice healing by the power of Allāh ta'ālā (﷾).

45. Impotence

- Beat 7 eggs from the country and mix them with 1 teaspoon of black seed powder. Eat this every day for 1 month.

46. General Weakness

1. Grind 1 cup of black seed and 1 cup of fenugreek. Mix them with amber oil and honey.

2. This mixture is eaten like jam with whole wheat bread every day at any time of day.

47. Weak Appetite

1. Before eating, take 1 teaspoon of finely ground black seed and chew it properly.

2. Drink 1 cup of cold water with a couple of drops of vinegar and you will notice the difference. Beware of bitna (excessive eating).

48. Lethargy and Laziness

1. Drink 1 cup of orange juice with 10 drops of black seed oil on an empty stomach every day for 10 days.

2. You will soon notice how vital and content you will become, inshā'a-llāh (ﷻ).

3. We recommend you do not go back to sleep after Fajr prayer (the pre-dawn prayer). Get used to sleeping after ʿIsha prayer (the evening prayer) and frequently remember Allāh taʿālā (ﷻ).

49. Mental Activation and Faster Memorization

1. Boil some peppermint and sweeten the tea with honey.

2. Add 7 drops of black seed oil and drink this tea warm at any time of day.

3. Soon you will notice the blossoming of your intelligence and your ability to memorize.

The Medicinal Use of Figs

1. Underweight

1. Bring to a boil 7 chopped figs and 1 teaspoon of anise in enough water to cover them.

2. Drink 1 cup of this mixture on an empty stomach in the morning and 1½ hours before dinner.

2. Poisoning and Toxicity

- Eat figs with walnuts as lunch.

Another Remedy

- Mix figs with common rue (Ruta graveolens) and eat the mixture on an empty stomach.

3. Activating Memory

- Mix together 3 figs, almonds and pistachios and eat them for lunch.

4. Balancing the Gastro-Colic Response

1. Mix chopped figs with a little bit of soda ash (sodium carbonate) and water.

2. Cook on low heat.

3. Take 1 teaspoon of the mixture on an empty stomach.

5. Lung Diseases

1. Boil 7 figs and ½ cup of fenugreek in water.

2. Strain and drink.

6. Getting Rid of Gas

1. Mix together 7 chopped figs, 1 teaspoon of common rue and 1 teaspoon of anise.

2. Cook in water and then drink 1 cup of the liquid after cooling.

7. The Spleen

1. Soak 1 kilogram of figs in apple cider vinegar for 9 days, making sure the vinegar covers the figs completely.

2. Eat the figs and drink the liquid.

3. Also, soak a bandage in this mixture and place on top of the ribs on the left side of the body where the spleen is located.

8. Skin Disorders: Vitiligo, Warts, etc.

1. Mix and grind the following ingredients together:

    7 figs
    ½ cup of wheat or barley flour
    ½ cup of fenugreek
    ½ cup of olive oil

2. Mix everything properly and add some more olive oil until the dough becomes smooth like cream. Apply this to the infected area.

To remove warts do the following:

1. Chop some wood from the fig tree and burn it until it has almost turned into coals.

2. Cauterize the warts carefully and they will totally disappear.

9. Gingivitis and Cavities

1. Chop some figs and mix them with wild fig "milk"[22] and soda ash (sodium carbonate).

2. Mix it together properly and apply the mixture to the infected gums and teeth every day in the morning and evening.

10. Skin Ulcers

1. Burn 7 figs to ashes.

---

[22] The fig tree produces a liquid that resembles milk instead of resin.

2. Mix the ashes with 1 teaspoon of olive oil and apply the mixture as an ointment to the ulcers.

11. Rheumatism, Gout and Thick Tumors

- Eat a large amount of figs, dried or fresh, for lunch on a regular basis.

12. Dermatitis and Rashes from Bed Bugs

1. Blend together 7 figs, 3 egg yolks and 50 grams of beeswax until the mixture is creamy and soft.

2. Apply it to the infected surfaces.

13. Internal Ulcers and Vaginal Discharge

To help avoid inflammation and ulcers, prepare the following remedy.

1. Mash 2 figs and mix them well with 1 teaspoon of honey.

2. Smear some of the mixture on a piece of wool and use it as a vaginal suppository.

3. Repeat this treatment until the infections are gone.

14. Epilepsy, Insanity and Obsession

1. Cook ripe or dried figs with black seed in little water.

2. Eat the figs and drink the liquid after adding 7 drops of black seed oil to it.

15. Abdominal Pain

1. Chop 3 figs and mix with them with common rue.

2. Cook the mixture properly in little water.

3. Eat after the mixture has softened.

16. Cracked Heels

1. Extract the sap of the fig tree and preserve it in a glass flask.

2. Apply it to your cracked heels in the morning and evening.

17. Severe Constipation
1. Mix together fresh or dried figs with 1 teaspoon of olive oil.

2. Take the mixture on an empty stomach in the morning and evening until the constipation is over.

18. Vitality and Strength
Eat reasonable amounts of figs, whether they are fresh or dried, instead of lunch. Do not excessively eat figs, for they will block your appetite. People suffering from gastric inflammation should not eat more than 6-7 figs per day, because fig seeds might damage the healing process of the stomach.

19. Respiratory System Conditions (including Sore Throat, Tracheitis and Whooping Cough)
1. Slice 20 figs in half.

2. Soak the halves in ½ liter of hot water for 12 hours.

3. Drink the liquid in the morning and evening.

20. Pharyngitis
• Take the remedy for the respiratory system as described above and in addition, gargle with the liquid at night and in the morning.

21. Lazy Bowel Syndrome (Infrequent Bowel Movements)
1. Slice 3 fresh or dried figs in half.

2. Dip them in olive oil and then cover them with slices of black lime (dried lime) for a whole night.

3. Eat the figs in the morning.

22. Minor Burns

1. Mash a suitable amount of figs (according to the size of the area to treat) until they are smooth and soft.

2. Apply the paste to the burns, cover them with gauze and carefully tie something around the gauze to keep it in place.

23. Abscessed Tooth and Mouth Ulcers

- Slice figs in half and place them on the infected areas.

24. Visible Tumors

1. Boil figs with a little water on low heat until they totally soften.

2. Add dried goat scybala (excrement) and mix properly.

3. Apply the mixture to the tumors.

25. Sore Throat

1. Cook figs and soft pomegranate peel in water.

2. Gargle with the liquid produced.

26. Itchiness

3. Cook some figs with mustard foam.

1. Rub it on the itchy areas.

27. Smallpox, Palpitations and Low Body Temperature

1. Blend together 5 figs, 7 grams of coriander and 20 grams of fennel seeds.

2. Take this on an empty stomach daily until the condition is healed.

28. Kidney Tumors

1. Boil 5 figs in a little water and then add ½ cup of honey.

2. Apply close to the infected area and place a bandage over it.

29. Inflamed Cornea

1. Mix 1 tablespoon of fig sap and 1 tablespoon of honey.

2. Drop it into the infected eye several times in the morning and evening.

30. Chronic Cough (lasting more than 8 weeks) and Chest Pain

1. Slice 20 figs in half and soak them in 1 liter of hot water for 12 hours.

2. Stain and drink the liquid.

*   This recipe can be also used for lung tumors.

31. Thirst, Kidneys and the Bladder

*   Eat fresh figs frequently.

32. Diuresis

1. Prepare a fig compote: immerse whole pieces of dried fig in water until the figs have softened.

2. Drink the syrup in the morning before breakfast on an empty stomach.

33. Blood Purification

1. Soak the following in warm water for 12 hours: 5 figs, 7 dates and ¼ cup of raisins.

2. Take this remedy as a purifier, as well as for its nutritional value.

34. To Cleanse the Stomach and Empty the Bowels

*   Frequently eat either dried or fresh figs on an empty stomach. Preferably, eat them immediately after they have been picked off the tree.

35. Pimples / Acne

- Thoroughly mix salt and fig sap and apply it to the acne.

36. Hemorrhoids

1. Boil 50 grams of calf kidneys and 50 grams of finely chopped figs until the mixture is soft and smooth.

2. Mix it with finely ground black seed and little sugar.

3. Prepare rectal suppositories from the mixture.

37. Common Cold

1. Bring the following to a boil in water: 5 figs, dill, celery and thyme.

2. There should be 10 times more water than figs, dill, celery and thyme. Boil until the water has reduced to ¼ its original quantity.

3. Strain and drink.

38. To Regulate the Menstrual Cycle

1. Boil 30 grams of fig leaves in 1 liter of water on low heat for 5 minutes.

2. Strain and drink the liquid after it has cooled.

- You can drink this several times a day.

39. Treatment for Painful Menstruation

1. Crush some dried fig leaves into a powder.

2. Add 1 teaspoon of this powder to 1 cup of milk (or yogurt) and mix.

3. Drink this several times a day for several days.

The Medicinal Use of Chamomile

Intestinal Disorders and Inflammation

1. Boil ½ teaspoon of chamomile in 1 cup of water until it is concentrated.

2. Drink for long durations in equal doses.

Abdominal Pain

1. Boil 40 grams of chamomile with 30 grams of lemon balm (Melissa officinalis).

2. Add 2 teaspoons of this mixture to water and drink.

Cramps and Diarrhea in Children

- Drink 1 cup of boiled chamomile. For each cup of water, use ½ teaspoon of chamomile.

Gastric Ulcers (Stomach Ulcers)

1. Drink boiled chamomile (as recommended in the previous treatment).

2. Lie down on your back for 5 minutes and then on your right side for another 5 minutes.

3. Lie on your stomach for 5 minutes and then finally lie on your left side for 5 minutes.

Tonsillitis and Mouth Ulcers

- Gargle with boiled chamomile 3 times a day until the ulcers / infections are gone.

The External Use of Chamomile

Rheumatism, Nerve Pain, Dermatitis

1. Prepare a warm poultice of chamomile and place it on the infected or painful area.

2. Tie a piece of gauze around the treated area carefully to keep the poultice in place.

Conjunctivitis, Ulcers, Eczema and Scabies

- Prepare a compress of boiled chamomile and place it on the area to be treated for 10 minutes, 3 times a day.

Nasal Congestion, Common Cold and Urinary Tract Infection

1. Gargle with boiled chamomile water.

2. Also, do a chamomile steam: boil chamomile flowers in water and inhale the steam for several minutes.

Migraines and Headaches

1. Soak your feet in boiled chamomile for 10 minutes before bedtime.

2. Then, dry your feet properly and wear wool socks.

3. Drink 1 cup of boiled chamomile and then go to sleep.

Hair Brightener for Blondes

Chamomile flowers provide a brighter hair color for blonde women.

1. Wash your hair with boiled chamomile (1 teaspoon for every 1 liter of water) 2 or 3 times a week.

- This is better than artificial shampoos that lighten or brighten your hair.

The Medicinal Use of Parsley

Parsley is a green herb rich in calcium, phosphorus and iron. It is a good source of vitamins A, B, B_7 (biotin), and C. It is beneficial, as well, for the proper functioning of the thyroid and adrenal glands. Here are the most important benefits of parsley:

- Smallpox
- Hepatitis
- Menstrual pain
- Kidney health
- Painful urination
- Breast milk production

Mix parsley juice with any kind of fruit juice and drink 2 cups a day.

To Remove Kidney Stones

1. Boil 1 teaspoon of parsley seeds in 1 cup of water.

2. Drink 1 cup in the morning and 1 cup in the evening.

Arteriosclerosis, Sprains and Eye Infections

1. Roast parsley leaves and then mash them.

2. Put them in a poultice to place on the infected area.

Skin Blemishes and Freckles

- Prepare a skin cleanser with about 10 grams of parsley leaves, 10 grams of parsley roots and about ¼ cup of water.

- Boil them and then apply the liquid to the skin.

The Medicinal Use of Date Palm Shoots

Ancient physicians claimed that palm shoots could enhance a man's sexual ability if taken with honey; they are also helpful for female infertility (see below):

- Mix date palm shoots with honey and take 3 teaspoons a day for 3 days.

- Besides following the above procedure, you can apply date palm shoots topically before sleep. This helps infertile women because the shoots contain sex hormones and they stimulate the sexual glands. These findings were tested by many scientists and are found to be true—and Allāh (ﷻ) knows best.

The Medicinal Use of Lupin

Scabies and Pimples

- Mix finely ground lupin powder with honey to apply to the infected areas as an ointment.

- You can use lupin oil instead of the powder and honey. When doing so, apply it directly to the infected areas.

Other Advantages

It has been proved scientifically that lupin contain about 20% protein, cellulosic fibers and lenolic acid from calcium and phosphorus; lupin serves in cases of neurasthenia. Experiments have proven that there is a hormone in lupin that is a cerebrospinal gland extract. This extract is a powerful tonic for uterine contractions.

Recent lab experiments show that lupin powder is an alkaline that helps moisturize the skin, as well as healing many skin diseases. It is also known to eradicate kidney stones and gallbladder stones. It is also a treatment for difficult or painful urination. Moreover, lupin helps reduce hypertension and blood sugar levels for diabetics.

The Medicinal Use of Strawberries

Strawberry juice is used to treat schistosomiasis (a type of parasitic infection), digestive disorders, cases of coughing and whooping cough. Ancient medical practitioners confirmed that strawberries have many advantages in healing inflammation and various types of ulcers (i.e. mouth sores and sore throat). The following treatments are some examples of strawberry's benefits:

Fever, Measles and Sore Throat
- Gargle with strawberry juice 3 times a day and drink strawberry juice.

Diarrhea and Intestinal Parasites / Worms
- Boil strawberry roots and drink 1 cup daily on an empty stomach in the morning.

Stomatitis,[23] Cryptitis,[24] and Digestive Disorders
1. Boil strawberry flowers and fresh leaves in water. Strain and drink the liquid.

2. Also, eat fresh strawberries, for they have a sterilizing effect.

Impotence and Diabetes
- Eat fresh strawberries frequently and drink strawberry juice 3 times a day.

Adolescent Acne and Skin Softener
1. Prepare a facial mask: mash strawberries, apply the mash to the affected areas and leave it on for 20-30 minutes.

2. Wash your face with warm water and then rose water.

3. Repeat this twice a week.

---

[23] Inflammation of the mucosal lining of any of the structures in the mouth.
[24] Inflammation of an intestinal crypt.

The Medicinal Use of Tamarind (Indian Dates)

Tamarind contains abundant minerals, vitamins, proteins, fats, carbohydrates and citric acid. According to Mecca's vendors of herbs and spices, tamarind is a remedy for intestinal problems and a solution for intestinal parasites. The following are prescriptions for specific diseases:

Constipation, Intestinal Disorders and Laziness

- Soak tamarind in water and then drink the liquid. It acts as a gentle laxative that helps refresh and cool at the same time. The dosage is unlimited.

Acidosis[25] and Toxic Blood

- Given the existence of various acids and minerals in tamarind, regularly drinking liquid in which tamarind has been soaked increases the blood's pH level, which helps bring it into balance. It also purifies the blood of toxins.

To Lower Body Temperature and Treat Fevers Caused by Certain Abdominal Diseases

- Meccans use tamarind to refresh and cool the body, as well as to purify it from germs because it contains natural antibiotics.

Other Advantages

The latest scientific research has proven that tamarind contains antibiotics that are able to eradicate many types of bacterial dynasties. It is clear, therefore, why many pharmaceutical companies add liquid extract of tamarind to some of their drugs, especially to children's medicines and medicines that reduce fever.

---

[25] Increased blood acidity.

The Medicinal Use of Arugula

Arugula is a green herb rich in necessary vitamins and nutrients for the human being. This herb is vital for the renewal of red blood cells. It is also a cure for many cases of fatigue, suffering and pain.

Arugula has been proven to be most efficient in deactivating toxic substances in the body. It also reduces phlegm, eliminates kidney stones and reduces blood sugar levels (thus, it is good for diabetics).

1. Difficult or Painful Urination, Painful Menstruation, Pimples, Adolescent Acne

1. Boil 1 bundle of arugula and 1 large chopped onion.
2. Drink ½ cup in the morning on an empty stomach and ½ cup at night before bedtime.
3. Eat fresh arugula leaves regularly with meals.

2. Bleeding Gums, Indigestion, Induced Phlegm in the Respiratory System, Rheumatoid Arthritis, Pain, Diabetes and Tuberculosis

- Drink arugula juice 3 times a day.

3. Fragile Hair and Hair Loss (especially after dieting)

1. Mix arugula juice with rose petals.
2. Apply the mixture on the scalp and hair for 3 minutes and then wash it out.

4. For the Rapid Healing of Skin Ulcers

1. Mix together ground dried arugula leaves, 1 medium onion, strawberries and flax oil.
2. Strain the mixture and then use the liquid as a topical ointment for ulcers.

The Medicinal Use of Yellow Carrot

Yellow carrots are considered a tremendous source of vitamin A because they contain calcium in a form that is easily absorbed and digested. Yellow carrots are very beneficial in the following cases:

Toddler's Diarrhea (chronic diarrhea in kids 6 months–4 years old)

- Add carrot juice or carrot powder to a baby's milk and this remedy will help stop the diarrhea.

Intestinal Parasites, Seizures of Hepatitis and Diabetes

- Drink either fresh yellow carrot juice or the water from boiled carrot husk peels.

Wounds, Ulcers and Eczema

- Use the core of the yellow carrot topically on the affected area and place a bandage over it to keep the carrot in place. This will help boost the healing process of the skin.

Bruises, Arthritis and Mild Cuts

1. Boil yellow carrot leaves in some water.

2. Prepare them as topical bandages to place on the infected areas twice a day.

The parts of the yellow carrot used for the treatment of many diseases are the fruit, the seeds and the leaves. The most beneficial part of the yellow carrot is the seeds. They help treat cases of dropsy and they bring relief from colic pain. Carrot seeds facilitate the generation of urine, benefit the menstrual cycle and strengthen sexual ability. Cooking carrots with sugar helps heal leg and food disorders. Yellow carrot juice regulates the healthy function of the thyroid and protects it from nervous system disorders. In addition, its juice is helpful in eliminating intestinal parasites and worms and it also reduces blood sugar levels. It has additional advantageous effects for liver disease and it serves as a preventive treatment for kidney stones.

Lately, research in this field has proven the efficacy of yellow carrots in totally healing diarrhea and gastrointestinal ulcers. Its husked peels help cure many dermatological diseases when used as poultices. Finally, its core helps prevent seizures accompanied by some of the above-mentioned diseases (i.e. epilepsy).

The Medicinal Use of Nutmeg

For Internal Use
Nutmeg is mainly used as one of the most stimulating spices for the digestive system. Its extract is added to some types of medications and tablets in order to improve their taste. Nutmeg is typically important for activating the digestive system and eradicating intestinal gases.

For External Use
Nutmeg oil is used as a topical ointment for massaging the body. It strengthens the vision and helps activate digestion, as well as fortifying the functioning of the liver and spleen. It prevents nausea and stops respiratory phlegm if taken with honey. Its oil is also used in perfume production. It is also well-known for its treatment of rheumatism. However, it is important to remember that consuming large amounts of nutmeg may cause many nervous system and sexual disorders.

The Medicinal Use of Sycamore

(Acer pseudoplatanus)

Sycamore is used to treat many medical conditions, which include the following:

Gastroenteritis (Flu or Stomach Virus), Abdominal Bulges and Constipation

- Eat ripe, fresh sycamore fruit and drink 1 cup of its juice before breakfast on an empty stomach.
- Use sycamore sap as a topical ointment and sterilizer, especially for gastroenteritis and excessive stomach gas.

Gingivitis and Flaccid Gum Disease

- Chew sycamore fruit and keep chewing it for as long as possible. Also, gargle with its juice to enhance the treatment.

Psoriasis, Herpes, Wounds and Ulcers

- Use slices of sycamore fruit in poultices and then place them on the infected areas.
- Use sycamore sap as a topical ointment and sterilizer.
- Besides treating gum diseases, sycamore is most efficient in treating liver diseases, dermatological diseases, as well as scorpion and snake bites.

The Medicinal Use of Fenugreek

Cough, Flu, Chest Pain and Difficult or Painful Urination

1. Boil fenugreek and drink a cup of its tea every morning on an empty stomach.

2. Or, take 1 teaspoon of fenugreek powder with honey 3 times a day.

Sore Throat, Bladder Pain, Gastroenteritis, Hemorrhoids, Constipation, Underweight and Sexual Impotence

1. Drink boiled fenugreek.

2. Also, cook fenugreek seeds properly in some water and eat 2-3 cups daily.

Gastric Ulcers and Peptic Ulcers (Gastrointestinal Ulcers)

- Mix fenugreek powder with vinegar and take 3 teaspoons daily.

Epilepsy

- Frequently drink boiled fenugreek and eat its seeds. This helps treat epileptic seizures.

The Medicinal Use of Chickpeas

In ancient medicinal recipes found in Mecca, chickpeas were used as a stomach laxative, to generate urine and to increase sexual vitality. In Arab medicine, chickpeas are considered an excellent food for the lungs. They clear the voice and remove hepatitis and spleen disorders, as well as kidney and gallbladder stones. Chickpeas are used in the treatment of the following:

Difficult or Painful Urination, Painful Menstruation, Kidney and Liver Weakness

1. Soak chickpeas for several hours.

2. Strain and drink the liquid.

3. Also, eat 3 teaspoons of chickpeas or its powder daily.

Shortness of Breath, Lung Diseases and the Common Cold

1. Roast chickpeas and add 1 teaspoon of them to 1 cup of yogurt.

2. Every morning and evening before bedtime, eat 1 cup of this on an empty stomach.

Cases of Jaundice

- Boil chickpea roots in some water properly. Drink 3 cups of the liquid a day.

Scabies and Ulcers

- Mix chickpea powder with honey and apply it as an ointment on the infected area twice a day.

The Medicinal Use of Common Mallow
(Malva sylvestris)

Common mallow leaves are used to treat many medical conditions, as follows:

For External Use

Dermatitis and Anal Ulcers
- Boil mallow leaves and use them as bandages on the infected areas.

Uterus Congestion and Vaginal Infections
1. Soak mallow leaves in ammonia and then strain.
2. Use the liquid as a vaginal cleanser, which will also help relieve pain.

Burns and Skin Swelling
- Grinding mallow leaves and olives is a very efficient way to treat burns and skin swellings.

Hemorrhoids
- Grinding mallow leaves with salt helps to treat hemorrhoids.

Breast Milk Production
- When eaten by a breastfeeding mother, mallow leaves will grant greater milk production, in addition to relieving coughs.
- Mallow flowers treat the kidneys and gallbladder when boiled and drank, and Allāh taʿālā (ﷻ) knows best.

The Medicinal Use of Carob

To treat Rheumatism, High Body Temperature and Gastroenteritis

1. Drink 1 cup of carob juice every 4 hours.

2. Soak some carob and drink the liquid to help reduce a high temperature and soften the stomach, as well as generate urine.

Carob is most beneficial in treating the common cold, anal infections, digestive disorders, rheumatic diseases and gastroenteritis. It is helpful for diabetics and tuberculosis patients. It is also used as a treatment for many gynecological diseases and to revive the heart and lungs. If it is mixed with yogurt and honey after it is boiled and strained, it becomes a tremendous remedy for constipation and difficult or painful urination. It is also a wonderful stomach cleanser and intestinal cleanser from parasites; in this case, drink one cup four times a day.

The Medicinal Use of Castor Beans

For Internal Use

Indigestion, Bacterial Gastrointestinal Infections, Constipation and Respiratory Phlegm

- Take 1 teaspoon of castor oil day after day until Allāh ta'ālā (﷾) grants you a full recovery, by His will.

To Relieve Rheumatic and Arthritic Pain, and Difficult or Painful Urination

1. Boil some castor leaves and flower petals and then strain.

2. Drink 1 cup of this liquid on an empty stomach every morning.

For External Use

To Remove Warts, Skin Blemishes and Scabies

- Wash the infected areas with soap and water and then apply some of the castor oil as an ointment.

To Remove Tumors, Infections and Breast Pain

- Mix equal amounts of castor oil and vinegar and use as a topical ointment before bedtime.

Headaches, Complicated Skin and Skin Structure Infections

1. Use castor tree leaves as bandages for the first day's treatment.

2. Then, apply castor oil as a topical ointment on the areas to treat.

3. Repeat as necessary.

Favus,[26] Fragile Hair and Skin Reddening

- Apply castor oil on the infected areas once a day.

---

[26] A fungal disease, usually affecting the scalp, characterized by yellow, circular crusts grouped in patches.

The Medicinal Use of the Mustard Plant

White mustard has many benefits and its use has resulted in remarkable outcomes in the treatment of many medical conditions. The most important are:

Weak Heart Muscle, Lung Infections and Gout

- Prepare a topical or full-body bath: add an average of 200 grams of mustard powder to a bath, after boiling properly.

Stomatitis, Tonsillitis and Sore Throat

1. Add 3 teaspoons of mustard powder to 2 cups of water and boil.

2. After the mixture is cool, gargle frequently.

Headaches, Gastric Ulcer Pain, Poor Circulation and Lung Congestion

1. For the treatment of these medical cases, prepare a poultice: mix mustard powder in warm water until it becomes a consistent paste.

2. Spread the paste evenly (1 centimeter thick) on a piece of cloth.

3. Place the poultice directly on the area that needs treatment (on the skin) and leave it there for 15-30 minutes.

   For instance, if you have a headache, place the poultice on the back of the head. In you have gastric ulcers, place the poultice above the stomach. For lung congestion and difficulty breathing, as well as poor circulation, place the poultice on the back. Place the poultice on the neck and throat area if you have a sore throat.

Mustard can be very helpful in cases of rheumatism and arthritis. Research has proven that mustard is a wonderful sterilizer and that

40 drops of it in 1 liter water is enough to turn the water into a medical sterilizer for the skin. In terms of preventing disease, mustard prevents cerebral palsy, arteriosclerosis and hypertension. It is enough to eat 2 mustard seeds in order to eradicate gastrointestinal gases. Generally, as well, mustard is quite advantageous for an intrinsically weak heart muscle and arteriosclerosis patients.

The Medicinal Use of Lettuce

Lettuce has essential nutrients that are extremely beneficial for the nervous system and muscles. The green leaves of lettuce are the most important part of this plant, for they contain certain substances that serve as a tonic and add vitality to the body. The most important of its treatments are as follows:

Chronic Constipation

- Eating lettuce is one of the most effective treatments for this disease, for lettuce contains dietary fiber that helps the intestines to function naturally.

Impotence and Infertility in Both Women and Men

- Eat fresh lettuce daily.

- This can help in cases of gout, gallstones and infertility, as well as erectile dysfunction. Frequently consuming lettuce may cure these diseases.

Complicated Skin and Skin Structure Infections, Skin Reddening and Painful Burns

1. Place lettuce leaves on the infected areas to cool them and relieve the pain.

2. This treatment also helps in removing skin tumors and infections; in this case, repeat the treatment twice a day.

Lettuce effectively quenches the thirst, reactivates the liver and stops nausea. Lettuce is quickly digested and it prevents excess stomach heat. Also, eating lettuce with vinegar is a powerful appetite stimulant, and it also generates urine. It strengthens eyesight and increases the level of fertility. In addition, its leaves contain a substance that absorbs unpleasant body odors. One of its most significant medical uses is that it adds moisture to the stomach, relieves cough, prevents constipation, is resistant to acidity and its seeds are used a tranquilizer with a sedative effect that causes sleeping.

The Medicinal Use of Ammi[27]

For Internal Use

Hepatitis Pain, Urinary Retention and Schistosomiasis (a Type of Parasitic Infection)
- Boil dried ammi seeds and drink 1 cup in the morning and evening.

Gallbladder Pain, Renal Colic and Gastrointestinal Muscle Spasms
- Boil ammi powder and drink 1 cup in the morning and evening.

Difficulty Breathing, Whooping Cough, Asthma, Chest Pain
1. Boil ammi powder and drink 1 cup in the morning and evening.

2. Also, boil ammi roots in water, strain, and drink 3 cups of the liquid a day.

For External Use

Chronic Skin Infections, Vitiligo and Psoriasis
- Apply an extract of ammi leaves as a topical ointment on the infected areas 3 times a day.

Because of the medical substance in this plant, it is considered a remedy for cases of trachea and ureter muscle spasms. In addition, it is a cure for biliary diseases and intestinal problems. It also dilates the blood vessels, especially the cardiovascular veins and the urinary tract. Research has proven that ammi can be used to treat vitiligo, psoriasis and alopecia by Allāh ta'ālā's will (ﷻ).

---

[27] Ammi is a genus of 3-6 species of plants in the Apiacae family.

The Medicinal Use of Peach

Constipation in Adults and Children

1. Boil peach leaves and strain.

2. Drink the liquid to treat constipation in adults.

- Simply drinking peach juice is enough for children with constipation.

Urinary Retention and Weak Bowel Movements

- Eat peaches for lunch.

- This also treats arthritis, gout and arteriosclerosis. It is preferable to eat peaches after meals, as well.

Peaches include vitamins A and C, carbohydrates, minerals (phosphorus, copper, sulfur, sodium and potassium), high levels of iron and calcium and in addition to organic acids. The organic acids in peaches efficiently treat urinary retention and they serve as a powerful laxative for the stomach and intestines. Peaches are also a cure for headaches, earaches, stomach worms and they enhance sexual energy. One of the peach's most important functions is treating arterial problems, rheumatism, constipation and gout; use dried peaches for these conditions.

The Medicinal Use of Galangal

(Blue Ginger or Laos)

For Internal Use

Indigestion and Excessive Stomach Gas
1. Boil dried galangal powder by adding 1 teaspoon of it to 1 cup of hot water.

2. Drink once a day.

For External Use

Inhale the steam of galangal powder boiled in water. Galangal is hot and dry, which helps open the pores of the skin; it is also an appetite stimulant, as well as a powerful digestive. It is known to heal sciatica as well as forehead and back pain. Drinking it diluted in sheep's milk helps restore your youthful strength, inshā'a-llāh (ﷻ).

The Medicinal Use of Cucumbers

Cucumbers contain large amounts of vitamin C in addition to moderate amounts of vitamins A and B. They also contain potassium, iron and silicon. The most significant of cucumber's remedies are:

Fevers, Neurological Disorders and Increased Thirst
- Chop up some cucumbers and add them to yogurt.

Indigestion, Constipation and Frequent Urination
- Eat fresh cucumbers consistently in the evening every day.

To Remove Body Odor and Activate Urine Production
- Consume large amounts of cucumbers continuously.

For the Treatment of Headaches
1. Slice rings of cucumbers and place them on the forehead and the temples.

2. Tie a piece of gauze to keep them in place and leave them on for 30 minutes.

For Softer and More Flexible Facial Skin and as a Facial Cleanser
1. In the evening, apply fresh cucumber juice to the face.

2. Leave it on until the morning. This serves a cosmetic, as well as a cleanser. Applying cucumber juice to your hair can also help repel insects.

The Medicinal Use of Doum

(Hyphaene thebaica, Gingerbread Tree or Thebaica)

Medicine men in Mecca know doum as a remarkable remedy for many diseases. Some of these diseases are bladder infections and difficult or painful urination. It is also a blood purifier. Doum is rich in carbohydrates, resins and essential alkalines. The following are what this plant is able to treat:

Fevers and Hypertension

1. Soak some doum fruit in water for several hours until the fruit is soft.

2. Drink the liquid and eat the fruit.

Another way to prepare this remedy

1. Crush the spongy cover of the doum until it becomes a powder.

2. Add 3 teaspoons of this powder to 1 cup of water and sweeten it with sugar.

3. Drink 4 cups daily.

Difficult or Painful Urination, Bladder Pain, Painful Fractures

- Prepare some doum using the method previously mentioned.

It is proven that doum is used to treat urinary retention and blood in the urine. It relieves pain from fractures and it strengthens the teeth. It smoothes the blood vessels and refreshes the body.

Recent research confirms that doum has great benefit when used to treat hypertension, for it is exceptional at lowering blood pressure.

The Medicinal Use of Thyme

For Internal Use

Chest Pain, Cough, Asthma, Congestive Hepatopathy,[28] Menstrual Pain, Bronchitis, Bladder Stones and Diarrhea

1. Boil thyme leaves in some water.

2. Strain, sweeten the liquid with honey or sugar, and then drink.

- This remedy applies to every one of the above mentioned diseases.

To Eradicate Oligochaetes (a Type of Worm) and Gas

1. Boil thyme leaves in water.

2. Strain and then drink the liquid or use the liquid in an enema.

Spasticity, Angina Pectoris and Fevers

- Boil thyme leaves in water, strain, and then drink the liquid.

For External Use

Conjunctivitis and Eye Strain

- Prepare small cloth sacs filled with hot thyme and place them topically on the eyes.

The Gallbladder

- Place small cloth sacs filled with hot thyme on the upper right side of the belly.

Toothache and Tonsillitis

1. Mix together 15 grams of thyme and 100 grams of water.

2. Boil and gargle with the liquid 3 times a day.

---

[28] Liver dysfunction due to venous congestion, usually of the right side of the heart.

Neurasthenia (Nervous Exhaustion) and Chronic Eczema

- Boil fresh thyme in water and then soak the whole body in it for 10-15 minutes daily.

Thyme contains thymol, which is considered one of the most powerful sterilizers that eliminates the deadliest microbes; it also eradicates intestinal worms and parasites.

In addition, thyme is rich in tannins and essential oils, as well as having many analgesic substances for pain.

Through the distillation of thyme's leaves and flowers, we get thyme oil, which is an essential volatile oil used in toothpaste. It is also a sterilizer for the nose and mouth. It is used to treat the common cold, cough and sore throat. Thyme oil is a cure for angina pectoris and spasticity diseases. It eliminates typhoid and dysentery microbes.

The Medicinal Use of Saffron

For Internal Use

To Relieve Pain from the Common Cold, Whooping Cough and to Tranquilize the Nervous System

1. Boil saffron flowers with a little water.

2. Strain and drink 3 cups of the liquid a day (while it is still warm).

Indigestion, Urinary Retention and Liver Weakness

- Boil saffron in water.

- Strain and drink 1 cup of the liquid in the morning and another in the evening before bedtime.

For External Use

Gingivitis (Bleeding Gums)

1. Boil saffron in some water.

2. Strain and allow the liquid to cool.

3. Use it to gargle 3 times a day.

Complicated Skin and Skin Structure Infections and to Improve Skin Color

- Use saffron oil as a topical ointment; apply it to the infected areas as needed.

- Boiled saffron in water can also be used as a cleanser.

Rheumatic Pain and Arthritis

- Massage the painful areas with saffron oil daily.

- Another way to apply this remedy: add 1 gram of saffron powder to 3 cups of boiling water. Use the liquid for massaging the painful areas, as well.

To Dye the Hair and as a Hair Cosmetic
- Add some saffron powder to hair dye and mix to highlight the color.

In addition to these diseases, saffron can be used to treat other medical conditions. It strengthens the vision, the heart, the respiratory system and the stomach; it is a wonderful tranquilizer for the senses. It can treat spleen diseases and increase urine production and sexual desire. It also heals malignant ulcers. When saffron is added to 1 egg yolk and eaten, it activates the nervous system and helps treat urinary retention, stomach pain and neurological spasms. Gargling with saffron water helps cure gum infections in children. Its oil is very beneficial for arthritis.

The Medicinal Use of Ginger

(Zingiber officinale)

For Internal Use

Cough, Common Cold, Flatulence and Stomach Colic

1. Boil ginger, strain and sweeten the liquid with sugar.

2. Drink 3 cups a day to activate circulation and to help produce saliva.

- In cases of indigestion, cold and poor circulation, chew small amounts of ginger root.

- It is preferable to drink it hot because it warms the body and activates the stomach, the heart and the circulation, inshā'a-llāh ta'ālā.

To Remove Phlegm and for Strained Vocal Cords

- Drink hot boiled ginger tea, for it removes the sputum and stimulates the production of saliva, which will help cure strained vocal cords.

For External Use

Rhinitis (Inflammation of the Nose) and Sore Throat

- Gargle with ginger tea 3 times a day.

Continuous Sneezing

- Inhale powdered ginger through the nose (very small amounts).

The Medicinal Use of Olives

Olives are used in the treatment of the following conditions:

Constipation, Gallstones and Excess Secretion of Bile
- Take 1 teaspoon of olive oil every morning on an empty stomach.

Stomach Weakness, Fever and Gangrene
- Boil olive leaves and strain...

- Drink 1 cup of the olive leaf water on an empty stomach.

Tonsillitis and Infected Hemorrhoids
- Mash 3 olives and use them as a topical poultice.

Bleeding Gums
1. Boil olive leaves and strain.

2. Gargle using the liquid mixture 3 times a day.

Massaging the hair with olive oil helps prevent hair loss and softens it. It can also be used as a facial cosmetic and as a painkiller for arthritis, sciatica and backache, inshā'a-llāh (⚘).

The Siwak

(Twig from the Salvadora Persica Tree)

The Prophet Muḥammad (ﷺ), may the peace and blessings of Allāh (ﷻ) be upon him, said, "If it was not harder for my nation, I would have ordered them to use the siwak at every prayer." It is also recorded that he (ﷺ) said that if a person gets up at night for prayer, he should cleans his mouth with the siwak. According to Bukhārī, the Prophet Muḥammad (ﷺ) said, "The siwak is purifying for the mouth and is pleasing to the Lord." According to Muslim,[29] the Prophet Muḥammad (ﷺ) began to use the siwak as he entered his home.

Ibn Al-Qayyim (� الله) relates, "The best siwak are the twigs taken from the arak tree (Salvadora persica). One should not use twigs from unknown trees, for they may be poisonous." Also, one should not use it excessively, for it might remove your teeth's natural polish; using a siwak too frequently can also remove your teeth's protection from germs and acidic steam rising from the stomach. When used in moderation, the siwak cleans the teeth, prevents decay, removes unpleasant smells from the mouth, activates the tongue, helps digestion and purifies the brain.

The best way to use the siwak is by wetting it slightly with rose water. In addition to some of the advantages the siwak has, it tightens the gums, stops sputum, clarifies the sight, prevents cavities, activates the function of the stomach, clears the voice, helps digestion, stimulates reading and praying, expels sleepiness, pleases Allāh taʿālā (ﷻ), the angels (عليهم السلام) admire it, and it increases the scale of one's good deeds. It is likely to be used at any time, at prayer time, as one awakes from sleeping, and the moment mouth odor changes.

The best siwak are taken from the arak tree. The Prophet Muḥammad's siwak (ﷺ), may the peace and blessings of Allāh (ﷻ) upon

---

[29] An important collection of ḥadīth.

him, was from the arak tree. Usually, a siwak is extracted from the tree's roots. On other occasions, it is taken from twigs on the branches. The tree should be no less than 2-3 years old. The siwak is picked either dried or green. It has a very special smell and a spicy-hot taste, for it contains sinigrin, a substance found in mustard which is responsible its pungent taste.

The arak tree grows in hot, tropical regions and it is mainly found in valleys, but rarely in mountains. It is similar to the pomegranate tree. ʿAsīr in Jizan (Saudi Arabia) is one of the regions known to be rich in this kind of tree. Additionally, it is found in Mount Sinai, Upper Egypt, Sudan, Iran and East India.

Medical research and studies have confirmed that the siwak is rich in sterilizers, cleansers and that it tightens the gums. It prevents bleeding gums, mouth moldiness and it eliminates different germs.

The siwak contains tannic acid, which is an antidote to mold and diarrhea. This acid is also a popular sterilizer used in treatments for bleeding gums; it is used to support gum health and it is used in tooth cleansers. Tannic acid also heals mild cuts in the mouth and it prevents bleeding.

As for sinigrin, it is a form of glucose that results from the combination of mustard oil and grape sugar. A yeast called myrosin is used to decompose these substances back to their original components. People who use the siwak for the first time sense its spicy and hot taste. This is the effect of the sinigrin, which totally eradicates germs.

Barley

Barley is one of the most ancient plants humanity has ever known. It is the most ancient nutrition people have ever known, therefore, it was the first plant used in ancient medicine. The first person to use barley as a medication was the ancient Greek physician Hippocrates of Cos (460 BC – ca. 370 BC). He used to cook it and apply it to infections, as well as using it to treat many cases of fever.

In Egypt, barley juice is popular because of its great benefits; it has been used medicinally for many generations. The earliest Egyptians used barley juice to heal coughs and throat roughness, to produce urine, to cleanse the stomach, to quench thirst, to cool body temperature and to suppress curiosity. For these conditions, boil ground barley with 5 times its quantity in water. Strain and then drink the water as needed.

The Prophet Muḥammad (ﷺ), may the peace and blessings of Allāh (ﷻ) be upon him, used to advise his companions to drink barley water and to use barley. This was mentioned and quoted in many of his sayings, some of which are the following:

Ibn Mājah quoted from ʿĀ'isha (ﺭ), who said:

> The Prophet Muḥammad (ﷺ) used to prepare barley soup whenever one of his family members was suffering from malaise. He would say, "May their thirst be quenched and may they be pleased and happy, like when one washes dirt off his face with water." (ibn Mājah 3445)

In ʿĀ'isha's authentic sayings (ﺭ), it was recorded:

> Whenever one of her relatives died, the women assembled and then dispersed (returned to their homes) except for her relatives and close friends. She (ﺭ) would order that a pot of talbīna[30] be

---

[30] Talbīna is made by adding 1-2 tablespoons of 100% whole grain organic barley flour to 1½ cups of pure water. Cook on low heat for 10-15 minutes (optional: add

cooked. Then tharīd[31] would be prepared and the talbīna would be poured on it. ʿĀʾisha (◉) would say, "Eat of it, for I heard the Messenger saying, 'Talbīna soothes the heart of the patient and relieves him from some of his sadness.'" (Bukhārī 5690).

In other narrations of ʿĀʾisha (◉) she said:

> You should eat the beneficial thing that is unpleasant to eat (talbīna), meaning broth. If any member of the Prophet's family was sick, the cooking pot would remain on the fire until one of two things happened, the person either recovered or died. (ibn Mājah 3446)

ʿĀʾisha (◉) also said about the Prophet Muḥammad (◉), may the peace and blessings of Allāh (◉) be upon him:

> When people came to Him seeking a cure for a family member, claiming that the person had pain and did not desire food he would say, "Take talbīna and have the patient sip it." In other similar cases he would say, "I swear upon He who holds my soul (◉), that it (talbīna) cleanses the stomach the way one washes dirt from the face." (Mustadrak of Ḥākim 7455)

Barley contains protein, starch and minerals, such as iron, phosphorus, calcium and potassium. It is also rich in hordenine and multiengine, which are known to be essential alkaloids for the human body.

Barley extract is prescribed for lung diseases (such as tuberculosis), general weakness, children below the normal range of growth, gastrointestinal weakness, and kidney and bladder infections. As a remedy for these cases, boil 30-50 grams of barley in 1 liter of water. Let it simmer for 30 minutes. Strain and then drink the water.

---

milk or yogurt and sweeten with honey). Drink at least 1 cup daily. This may also be added to soup or any dish for flavor and as a thickener. Alternatively, you can substitute organic milk for the water.

[31] A dish prepared with meat and bread.

The same mixture can be used to clean festering wounds. The alkaloid hordenine can be extracted and injected under the skin or through drinking to treat diarrhea, dysentery and enteritis.

In cases of dermatitis, barley flour poultices can be used to treat the infected areas.

The Medicinal Use of Fennel

Fennel is an aromatic plant that reaches 1.5 meters in height. It has many branches and yellow flowers. Its seeds are grey and it has different names in other countries.

In ancient medicine according to Arab physicians, fennel helps clear the arteries, sharpen the vision, increase the production of breast milk and prevent glaucoma. Fennel benefits the menstrual cycle, the kidneys and the bladder; it serves as a painkiller and it dissolves gas. Inhaling its steam relieves headaches.

In modern medicine, fennel is known to contain vitamins A, B and C, as well as calcium, iron, phosphorus and potassium. In addition, it has an aromatic extract.

Its special features are: fluid production, strengthening, stimulating appetite, eliminates gas and intestinal parasites and stimulating the sexual glands. If it is given as a drink to children, it immediately tranquilizes them and puts them to sleep. The latter remedy is prepared by boiling fennel powder in 1½ cups of water and then adding some sugar.

This remedy also helps patients suffering from cough and asthma. Also, it is possible to give children this mixture for intestinal pain using an enema. A breastfeeding mother had better drink this mixture of fennel powder boiled in water in order to provide lots of milk for her infant. Additionally, this drink is the solution for a mild common cold and will totally discharge it.

Add dried fennel to heavy foods such as broad beans and common beans while cooking. This will make them more easily digested.

The Medicinal Use of Melon

The best melons are the dark yellow ones with a rough peel. They should be heavy, roundish and ribbed.

In ancient medicine, melons were prescribed for dropsy, jaundice and blocked arteries. They increase urine and feces production, they soothe and moisturize the skin, they remove moldiness, they dissolve kidney stones and they relieve the stomach.

In modern medicine, melons are sometimes used interchangeably with watermelons. This is due to the fact that melons contain a high percentage of water and they are high in carbohydrates (they can reach about 5%). However, melons have more vitamin C than watermelons.

It is true that melons are used in a way that is similar to watermelons when treating certain conditions that require a laxative and a remedy that is cooling and soothing to the body. Melons, however, are richer in iron, copper, sulfur, potassium, calcium and phosphorus.

Melons are significantly beneficial for the following conditions: anemia, constipation, hemorrhoids, low urine output and lack of bile secretion. Conversely, they are not used to treat diabetics, indigestion and enteritis.

Melons are used as a facial cosmetic, for they provide the face with a natural glow and softness; they are especially beneficial for dry skin disorders. The remedy for dry skin is: prepare a facial cleanser by mixing together equal amounts of distilled water, fresh milk (not boiled) and melon juice. Apply to the face as necessary.

Black Tea

Water absorbs many of tea's active ingredients when boiled or steeped for long time; this affects the concentration of some of its components. Many people believe that the more tea is boiled, the more of its stimulants we receive. However, the truth is that a few moments of steeping are enough to absorb large amount of caffeine. This is due to the fact that caffeine is easily dissolved in water. Boiling tea for a long time leads to the extraction of tannins, which do not dissolve well in water; large amounts of tannins can be very dangerous.

The most important features of tea are: tea is a stimulant, for it contains caffeine that stimulates certain nerve centers. Tea has also a positive effect on the heart, for it strengthens and increases the heart rate. This, in return, activates circulation. However, tea has a slight effect on urine production.

To conclude, tea is a beneficial stimulating drink when consumed in moderation, because 1 cup of tea has the equivalent of 1½ grains of caffeine.

Exceeding the normal amount of caffeine in the body will cause headaches and heart rhythm disorders. It takes 7 grains of caffeine, which can be found in 7-14 cups of tea, for these symptoms to occur. One hundred and fifty-five caffeine grains are enough to kill a human being. This means that 155 cups of tea can begin killing someone by causing poisonous heart rhythm disorders, difficulty breathing, loss of appetite, a yellowish pigmentation of the skin and indigestion. Constipation and indigestion occur due to the large consumption of tannins. Tannins are used to tan the skin. However, if tea is prepared in the correct way, one can avoid the extraction of tannins.

The Proper Way to Prepare Tea

1. One way to properly prepare tea is to pour boiling water on the tea leaves and let them steep for 5 minutes.

2. Strain and then drink.

If you boil tea, there a high risk of extracting the tannins. You know this has happened when the color of the tea turns from transparent gold to black.

It is important to note that it is preferable not make tea with metal utensils. Additionally, do not have tea while eating foods that contain iron or calcium. Tea will simply dissolve the essential minerals and vitamins. Finally, it is suggested to prevent children and the elderly from drinking tea or consuming a lot of it.

Date Palm Pollen

Date palm pollen is located at the top of the palm tree (its heart). The pollen is formed in small shapes that look like tiny fish. If they are opened, a thick white substance very similar to flour spreads out with a smell very similar to male semen. This is how male palm trees fertilize female palm trees.

This white pollen, when filtered, helps heal gallbladder infections, thirst, fever, diarrhea, bleeding and coughing up blood.

However, palm pollen has some disadvantages. It deactivates the stomach, especially for diabetics, and it is digested slowly. It may cause chest pain, stomach and kidney flu and urine retention. These conditions can be treated with celery and thyme. Its soft and mature pollen is used, in particular, to increase male and female sexual desire.

Allāh ta'ālā (ﷻ) mentions this pollen in the Qur'ān:

والنخل باسقات لها طلع نضيد

"And tall palm trees laden with clusters of dates." (50:10)

As well as:

وزروع ونخل طلعها هضيم

"...fields, palm trees laden with fruit..." (26:148)

These verses describe how generous Allāh (ﷻ) is for creating pollen, making the palm trees full of fruit.

Modern medicine has proven that 17% of pollen is sucrose, 22% protein and 54% calcium, in addition to high levels of vitamins B and C, phosphorus salts and iron.

It also well-proven that it gives tremendous strength to the body, for it is rich in oils and testosterone, which stimulates the ovaries and regulates the menstrual cycle.

Scientists have learned to extract a kind of protein from the pollen that is responsible of strengthening the capillaries in the human body and prevents their explosion. As a result, this will help prevent internal bleeding that affects hypertension and diabetic patients.

Tomatoes

Tomatoes are one of the most important vegetables on the table. They are rich in vitamins B and C and contain a smaller percentage of vitamins A and D. The tomato contains other nutrients and is comprised of 1.1% protein, 4.2% carbohydrates, 1.1% minerals, 0.6% fats and coloring and 1.6% cellulose.

One tomato provides an individual with one-third of his or her daily required amount of vitamin C.

Tomatoes are eaten fresh, cooked and their juice is drunk. However, when tomatoes are cooked, much of their nutrition dissolves.

People who suffer from stomach diseases, gastric acidity and enteritis are forbidden to consume tomatoes. Also, it is recommended that you remove the peel before eating a tomato, especially patients who have a weak stomach and inflammation of the rectum.

Tomatoes are prescribed for patients with rheumatism, bladder stones, gallbladder and kidney disorders, arthritis, stomach mold and constipation. For these conditions, tomatoes should be eaten fresh with their peels. This fruit is digested with no trouble; its nutrition is easily imparted to the blood and it travels in the circulatory system, carrying many essential needs for the human body.

Tomatoes can be used to remove calluses from the feet. This is done by soaking the infected foot in warm water for 10 minutes and then placing a slice of green, unripe tomato on the callus while the foot is still in water. After the treatment, cover the infected area with a piece of cloth and remove it in the morning. Repeat this remedy for five nights in a row until the callus is totally dissolved.

Sunflower (Helianthus annuus)

Sunflower is named "the eye of the sun" and "the slave of the sun" in Arabic. Indians used to consider it a sacred plant.

Sunflower seeds are very popular in markets today and they are entertaining snacks for many people. These seeds were used by ancient physicians to heal malaria, to produce urine and to dissolve sputum. Sunflower seeds are rich in protein, minerals and vitamins. They contain phosphorus and glycerin, which make them most beneficial in reducing cholesterol levels and preventing arteriosclerosis.

American and English dentists have noticed for many generations that eating sunflower seeds continuously creates healthy gums and teeth. This is because they contain phosphorus and calcium, as well as small amounts of fluoride, which strengthens the teeth and prevents decay.

Sunflower seeds contain a high proportion of essential oil. Seventy grams of this type of oil should be consumed every day, on average. Eating sunflower seeds before dinner gives you enough of the nutrients this oil provides.

Lentils

The legendary Antioch physician of the 11th century, Dāwūd al-Anṭākī (☀), mentions the following in his famous book *at-Tadhkīra* (*The Memento*),[32] "Lentils soothe high temperatures, dissolve fever, cure cough and lung pain. Swallow thirty grains to strengthen your digestive system. Lentil powder is beneficial for cauterizing and healing wounds. Use it to clean the body, for it purifies the skin and restores its natural color. Mixing vinegar, honey and egg whites with red lentils creates a good topical remedy for chronic skin tumors, dropsy and sagging skin. This plant burns up blocks in the lymphatic system."

However, lentils may cause vision and eye disorders; becoming addicted to lentils may result in cancer and leprosy, and even a pseudo-obstruction of the colon or hemorrhoids. Beware of cooking lentils with dried meat, for this can cause hard-to-cure illnesses, bloating and stomach gurgling.

Using lentils in a bandage, in addition to quince and coronet, resolves the common cold and conjunctivitis. If lentils are corrupted for one reason or another, it is possible to repair them and still be able to use them. This is done by simply boiling them in water with some vinegar and sesame oil.

Bitter lentils are known to have special benefits when used to heal itchiness and wounds, leaving no signs on the skin after it has healed. Moreover, if used to wash and clean the face along with watermelon seeds, they clear a yellowish pigmentation and add youth and redness to the skin.

---

[32] He was born in Antakia and died in Mecca in (1543-1599 C.E.). Dāwūd al-Antāki's *Tadhkirat ʾuli-l-albāb wa-l-jāmiʿa li-l-ajābu-l-ʿujāb* is a medical book popularly known as *Tadhkirat Dāwūd al-Antāki* or *Tadhkira*. The book was completed by his students and contains 1,712 drug entries (when the canon at the time had less than 800). It provides information on diseases, medicine, drugs and individual plants.

Lentils are also mentioned in the Holy Qur'ān when Allāh ta'ālā (ﷺ) says:

وإذ قلتم يا موسىٰ لن نصبر علىٰ طعام واحد فادع لنا ربك يخرج لنا مما تنبت قال أستبدلون الذي هو أدنىٰ الارض من بقلها وقثائها وفومها وعدسها وبصلها وضربت عليهم الذاه والمسكنة اهطوا مسرا فإن لكم ما سألتم بالذي هو خير

"Remember when you said, 'Mūsā (ﷺ), we cannot bear to eat only one kind of food, so pray to your Lord to bring out for us some of the earth's produce, its herbs and cucumbers, its garlic, lentils and onions.' He said, 'Would you exchange better for worse? Go to Egypt and there you will find what you have asked for.'" (2:61)

Imām Ibn al-Qayyim (ﷺ), may he rest in peace, relates the following about prophetic medicine, "There are many sayings attributed to our Prophet Muḥammad (ﷺ), may the peace and blessings of Allāh (ﷺ) be upon him, which are vividly untrue! Such as these, 'Seventy prophets sanctify it (the lentil),' and, 'It softens the heart,' and, 'It is the food of the righteous,' and, 'It is what the Jews desired and preferred over honeydew and quails (when they lived in the desert for years).'"

Al-Bayhaqī (ﷺ) narrates a story told by Ibn Isḥāq (ﷺ), "We asked Ibn Mubārak (ﷺ) whether the saying (about the lentil plant being sanctified by 70 prophets) is a true prophetic saying. He answered, 'No, this plant was not sanctified by any of the prophets; on the contrary, it is a bloating food and may harm some people! Who told you this?' They replied, 'Sālim ibn Sālim,' and he proceeded, 'Well, from whom did he hear it?' They replied, 'From you,' and he answered, 'Me?!'"

Today in modern medicine, lentils are agreed to be the richest among the nuts, beans and legumes. The French Department of Science in the twentieth century found that "cheese, lentils, beans, broad beans and peas are richer than beef in protein, carbohydrates and essential oils and fats."

Many people imagine that meat is the most nutritious food for the human body. Many chemical analyses prove this theory wrong, especially when considering an individual's functioning during the daily workday. People who physically work like farmers, laborers and postmen in villages or small towns perform better when relying on cheese and plants, not meat.

However, other research has shown that legumes are equal to meat, which is the source of many harmful and sometimes fatal acids and salts. The English Dr. Heige said that there is nothing more lethal to the human body than high concentrations of uric acid in the blood. This acid comes from foods like meat, legumes, coffee and tea. He advises people to avoid these foods totally, claiming that it is enough to consume green vegetables, cheese and fruit, for they contain all the nutrients required by a healthy human body.

Red lentils should not be prescribed for everybody unless they are healthy and make a substantial effort in their daily lives. It is forbidden to those who suffer from obesity, weak intestines, liver and kidney diseases, as well as gallbladder diseases. Red lentil peels fight constipation, produce urine and treat anemia, as well as preventing cavities. The remedy is to prepare poultices by boiling the peels of red lentils and then mashing them. The poultices are placed on the infected areas.

Juniper

Dāwūd Al-Anṭākī (☸) mentions the benefits of the juniper plant in ancient medicine in his famous book *The Memento*. He claims that it heals chronic cough, chest pain, weak stomach, gastrointestinal gas and pain, kidney disorders, frequent flow of liquids from the urethra, hemorrhoids and toxicity. One of its special features is that its smoke, when burned, repels insects. It is used in the making of bandages and as a cleanser. It stops excessive sweat and tightens up the body.

In modern medicine, juniper's fruits are known to have a gummy sap. This sap contains an essential oil that is remarkable at increasing appetite and urine production. This oil is also used to clean the urethra and in veterinary medicine it is used to soothe intestinal pain in animals.

It is used in the treatment of rheumatism. Simply boil the branches in water and wash your whole body with it. This treatment was proven to be effective in many cases where it was applied persistently and over a long period of time.

However, patients suffering from kidney disorders should avoid the use of juniper, whether for food or treatment, for it may be very harmful to them.

Use juniper oil or juniper sap to massage areas or joints suffering from rheumatism Do this two to three times a day and continue this treatment for several weeks. This remedy is prepared by mashing juniper flowers in a bowl of olive oil. This mixture should be preserved in a sealed container for ten days. Afterward, strain the mixture and use the oil. Similarly, one can prepare hair dye by adding alcohol instead of olive oil.

For the treatment of chronic skin diseases, boil juniper wood, strain and then drink the liquid. For the treatment of syphilis, boil twenty grams of juniper wood with a cup of water for ten minutes. Strain and drink several times a day.

A juniper fruit emulsion (also cooked) is taken in order to strengthen the immune system, especially for diabetics and those with excessive and/or copious urination suffering from poor appetite and general weakness. The same treatment helps to heal rheumatism. This emulsion is prepared by adding 1 teaspoon of mashed juniper fruit to one-quarter cup of very hot water. Mix properly and drink one-half cup daily.

Another way to prepare the same treatment using cooked juniper fruit: add fresh juniper fruit and four times its amount in water to a pot. Cook and stir frequently until the mixture becomes a paste. Take one teaspoon of this paste before eating twice a day.

Licorice

This is a perennial plant the Arabs call "sūs" and its roots are called "the origin of sūs," therefore, in Arabic it is named "'irqa-s-sūs." Its scientific name is Glycyrrhiza glabra.

This plant is described by Dāwūd Al-Anṭākī (⁂), "This plant is a herbaceous perennial. If it is planted in a certain place, it will be very hard to remove it. Its roots reach about ten cubits into the earth and become as thick as a man's thigh. Licorice flowers are between red and blue and the most beneficial part of the plant is its roots. The roots are at their best when they are fragile, yet coherent and sweet. Licorice root should be peeled before it is eaten because snakes rub their skins against the roots to clean them. It is also said that snakes use them to sharpen their vision. Eating licorice root beautifies the eyes and benefits coughs and lung diseases. It eradicates sputum totally, heals spleen and liver pain, dilutes thick urine, and heals and cleans hemorrhoids from waste products."

Greek physicians used to prescribe licorice root for the treatment of dry cough, asthma and thirst. Ibn Sīnā (⁂) mentioned in his book al-Qānūn (The Canon of Medicine)[33] that licorice root juice treats wounds, soothes and cleans the trachea, clears the voice, and quenches thirst. It helps in the treatment of stomach infections, difficult or painful urination, kidney ulcers, bladder ulcers and fever.

In modern medicine, studies and research on licorice root have found that this plant contains sugar, starch, glycerin and ospargen,[34] in addition to minerals like potassium, calcium, magnesium and

---

[33] Al-Qānūn fī-l-ṭibb is one of Ibn Sīnā's most famous works. Al-Qānūn provides a complete system of medicine according to the principles of Galen and Hippocrates. This book remained a medical authority until the early 19th century, setting the standard for medicine in Europe and the Islamic world.
[34] An amino acid that modern research shows to be important for increasing body strength.

phosphate. It consists of sex hormones and soap-like substances that form a foamy texture when drunk.

Given the fact that it consists of calcium oxalate,[35] licorice root can harm weak kidneys. Boiling licorice root in water and drinking the liquid is an effective medicine for indigestion and gastrointestinal ulcers. Much recent research has proven that this drink is activating and purifies the blood. One of licorice's ingredients is used in the treatment of Addison's disease (chronic adrenal deficiency), which puzzled doctors for a long time.

In order to heal constipation and to soothe the intestines, crush forty grams of licorice with forty grams of sulfur, forty grams of acacia, sixty grams of senna and two hundred grams of sugar cane. Mix the ingredients together and take one teaspoon every evening to soften the intestines. Take two teaspoons to loosen the stomach.

---

[35] A major component of kidney stones.

Ambergris (Grey Amber)

Ambergris is a solid and waxy substance produced in the digestive system of sperm whales. It is found in the whale's cecum enveloped by a yellow, orange or red liquid; it can also be found in the jaws of tiny sea creatures. This is ambergris; anything found that differs from than this description is not ambergris.

Ambergris is often found floating on the sea's surface near beaches in India, China, Japan, Africa and Brazil.

When this substance exits the animal's stomach, it is very soft. Chemically, it is 85% amber and 2.5% balsamic substance. It also contains a melted substance mixed with water and benzoic acid.

The Medicinal Use of Ambergris

Physicians see that ambergris strengthens the organs, enhances sexual performance and prolongs the lifespan. They also know that it has an effect on the heart and the nervous system. Part of it has been proven to benefit heart, pulse, brain and muscle functions, but the user can develop internal ulcers. In order to use it as a remedy, it requires a specific and careful prescription from a physician, for it may cause a very harmful outcome. Many doctors have succeeded in applying it in the treatment of dyspepsia (upset stomach) and chronic bronchitis.

Ambergris is an antiseptic; however, it can have a counterproductive result. Meaning, it may restore what medications have healed, as well as leading to the excessive fulfilling of desires (eating, sex, etc.). Many ambergris pastes and jams are being sold as food supplements or tonics. Actually, this is seriously dangerous for many reasons. People who buy these products to enhance their sexual abilities, for instance, will gain their strength back but with an excessive effect. This will temporarily lead to other problems, such as irritability. These side-effects soon dissipate, but an effect on the nervous system remains.

Even worse, if a person has a health condition he or she is unaware of and these products are taken, it may end their lives in several minutes.

Sweetgum

This tree has a balsamic sap and it grows in the areas surrounding the Mediterranean Sea and North America. Some Arab countries and Ethiopia have also successfully planted it.

The balsam is extracted from the tree by making incisions in the trunk. The sap, which is very similar to honey, begins to drop. The sap differs from area to area; it could be pure white or dark black with a very pleasant odor and a very spicy taste.

The active ingredients in sweetgum are essential oils, resins and cinnamic acid.[36] Authentic sweetgum activates the mucus membranes, helps treat chronic colds, strengthens the stomach and generates sweat.

There are ointments used to heal wounds that contain sweetgum sap. Arab physicians have mentioned that spicy and balsamic sweetgum is most effective in treating coughs and the common cold; it also eliminates sputum.

---

[36] So named because it is often obtained from the essential oil of cinnamon.

The Radish

In ancient medicine, Dāwūd Al-Anṭākī (ﷺ) said in *The Memento*, "Radishes purify the body from atherosclerosis[37] when mixed with water and honey; they clear the lungs and stomach, help digest food, expel gases and soften the stomach. Radish juice unblocks the vessels, and when added to honey and vinegar, it dissolves kidney stones. Radish roots make an effective remedy for certain liver disorders, reduced sexual performance, indigestion and vitiligo. This remedy is prepared by adding some radish root to four times the amount of turnip. Chop them all up and roast them with dough. Eat the mixture with honey. Indigestion is treated by simply drinking radish juice. As for skin color pigmentations, hair loss and alopecia, eat fresh radish and apply its juice to the infected areas. Deafness, arthritic pain, sciatica, gout and dropsy are treated by cooking radish in flower oil. Putting a few drops into an infected ear and using it to massage a painful area is very effective."

Ibn Sīnā (ﷺ) mentioned in *al-Qānūn*, "If bandages are prepared with radish, water and honey, even the worst of ulcers can be cured. A mixture of radish seeds and vinegar is beneficial for herpes; cooked radishes are an effective remedy for chronic cough and chymus.[38] Also, cooking radishes with vinegar and honey and then gargling with that liquid helps prevent diphtheria and increases the production of breast milk."

According to modern medicine, the radish helps heal colds, facilitates the production of urine and is a general cleanser. Drinking radish juice on an empty stomach dissolves bile acids, calms liver spasms, and helps indigestion, lung diseases, whooping cough and intestinal bacterial overgrowth.

---

[37] Build-up of fatty material in the blood vessels.
[38] Mechanical and chemical breakdown of fluids into the chest.

Given its composition of vitamins A and C, calcium salts, iron, iodine, sulfur and manganese, it efficiently treats skin diseases and anemia.

However, radishes are difficult to digest, for the peel contains essential. Therefore, patients who suffer from poor metabolism and a weak digestive system, as well as liver diseases, should avoid it.

Common Beans

Fresh, green or dried common beans are used in many foods. Green beans contain vitamins A, B and C and considerable amounts of minerals, such as calcium and phosphorus. They are also rich in chlorophyll. Dried beans, on the other hand, have protein, phosphorus, potassium, iron, calcium and vitamins B_2 (riboflavin) and C.

For medical use, green bean roots contain a substance called inositol (cyclohexane), which has a significant function in certain biological processes within the human body. Fresh green beans help renew white blood cells and treat heart disease, hypertension and indigestion. When consumed fresh, these beans are very soothing to the nerves. They generate urine, strengthen the liver and the spleen, treat growth hormone deficiency and help fatigue. They clear stones in the urinary tract, reduce excess albumin, support diabetics and increase the biomaterials in the body. All of these conditions are treated by drinking one-half cup of fresh green bean juice on a daily basis.

Dried beans are very nutritious and are better if consumed with their peels, for they contain essential enzymes. Dried beans are easily digested if cooked and eaten with other vegetables. They are usually prescribed for athletes, laborers and teenagers. However, they are prohibited for people who suffer from obesity, gastric cramps, indigestion or liver diseases. They are contraindicated for infants and pregnant women. To use them medically, cool them properly, mash them and then smear them in poultices to treat burns, skin infections and herpes.

The Broad Bean (Vicia Faba, Field Bean or Tic Bean)

Broad beans have been well-known since ancient eras; many amazing, legendary tales were told about them. In terms of nutrition, the nutritional value of broad beans equals that of other legumes. In modern medicine, it is found that broad bean flowers efficiently increase the production of urine, activate the digestive system, dissolve stones in the urinary tract, soothe kidney pain and stop vomiting. The remedy for these conditions is prepared by soaking 50-60 flower petals in two cups of very hot water. Strain and drink several times a day.

Boiling and drinking broad beans supports the treatment of bladder and kidney stones and infections and jaundice. If you have a weak stomach or indigestion, you are prohibited from eating broad beans in order to prevent these medical conditions from worsening.

Cinnamon

Cinnamon is taken from the bark of its sweet plant and it has a pungent taste and balsamic odor.

According to ancient medicine, cinnamon has a heating effect. It generates urine, clears the vision and removes warts and freckles. If it is mixed with honey, it can heal chronic cough, the common cold, kidney pain, urine retention, and it also dissolves sputum, enhances brain function, helps digestion, treats asthma, cleans the lungs, unblocks the liver vessels, strengthens the stomach, and treats diseases of the uterus (add it to honey and egg yolks).

Real cinnamon is simply called "cinnamon," and its peel is called "vanilla." This name is taken from the Latin word meaning "the little flute," which characterizes its quirky shape.

Cinnamon peel contains very effective essential oils, a pungent taste, lutein (an antioxidant), food coloring agents, starch, benzoic acid and chlorophyllin, which is a crystalline material extracted from carnations and cinnamon.

Cinnamon has also proven to be an effective stimulant for the heart, the stomach, the intestines, as well as the taste buds and mouth nerves. It increases sweat production, eases painful menstruation, helps the body to expel gas, increases appetite and supports digestion. Its essential oils provide it with its unique odor and taste; therefore, it is used in desserts and sweets. However, pregnant women should avoid cinnamon because it stimulates the womb, which might harm the fetus.

Cinnamon is used in the treatment of the common cold, cough, kidney pain, vocal cord nodules, lung sputum, and only some cases of vomiting and diarrhea due to the fact it contains a considerable amount of tannins. Therefore, it is preferable to drink diluted cinnamon tea so as not to harm the lining of the digestive system.

Cinnamon oil is extracted through distillation. Its color ranges from dark yellow to brown, and over the years it gets thicker and darker. This oil, called cinnamic aldehyde, is used for desserts and cosmetics; it has a unique odor and it should be preserved away from light and heat.

Cauliflower

Arab physicians have claimed that cauliflower eliminates gastrointestinal worms and parasites, dissolves tumors, heals wounds, cleans the spleen and the liver, unblock the vessels and dissolves kidney stones. By using cauliflower powder, one can treat cavities and tooth decay. Cauliflower and honey make a remedy that heals vocal cord disorders and constipation. Cauliflower treats dermatitis when applied to the infected areas.

In modern medicine, nutritionists claim that cauliflower, among other vegetables, contains a high amount of phosphorus, thereby enforcing body structure. Other scientists have mentioned that it helps in the decomposition of uric acid, which is a very necessary process in the human body. However, cauliflower is considered hard to digest, especially if cooked and fried with eggs. For this reason, if you have a weak stomach you should totally avoid consuming it.

Carnation

It is a small evergreen tree that has many crimson flowers. Carnation sprouts are characterized by greenish to reddish colors, which change to brown and become fragile-looking, like spikes.

Arab physicians used carnation and mentioned its many benefits. Taking about 5-6 grains of its powder (or several drops of its sap) and mixing it with sugar makes a great remedy for the nervous system; even if the nervous system has no issues, it will help it to function even more efficiently

If this remedy is used more frequently and in larger amounts, it soon leads to an overall stimulation of other body systems. It will stimulate the stomach, circulation and body tissues, and it will enhance organ function. Doctors discovered this fundamental feature of carnation and have prescribed it to patients with indigestion.

Carnation's unique odor stimulates the heart, strengthens the stomach and kidneys and the rest of the internal organs. It helps the digestive system, expels gastrointestinal gas, protects the gums, sharpens flavors and benefits the treatment of dropsy, for it heats and strengthens the kidneys.

Briefly, it is a remedy for all of the organs. It is even said that it can be used as an eyeliner to sharpen the vision, stop blurry vision and heal eye infections. It stops urinary incontinence. It also heats the uterus; if a woman wants to get pregnant, she just has to take an amount that weighs as much as a penny as the menstrual period ends.

In modern medicine, carnation is known to fight fever, sterilize and clean the stomach, heal ulcers and headaches, detoxify, alleviate tooth pain, decrease allergic infections, stimulate the heart and stomach and finally, stimulate the female reproductive system. These cases are treated with the following remedy: add a really small proportion of carnation powder to some sugar. Boil them in water and drink. This also helps a weak stomach, vomiting, diarrhea and fatigue. Carnation is prescribed as a wound sterilizer and a painkiller.

Carnation oil can be used to soothe a toothache: dip a piece of cotton in carnation oil and then clean the infected tooth with it. The pain will be gone in no time.

Stinging Nettle

This plant's stem is square-like with serrated heart-shaped leaves covering it. The stem has delicate filaments that hurt and irritate the skin if touched. Its flowers are tiny and green and they look like clusters hanging down.

This plant contains substances that infect the skin, produce urine and detoxify the blood. Another substance in stinging nettle is secretin, which is an enzyme that melts in water. In the past, this plant was used in industry and then it was discovered to be a very effective treatment for contaminated wounds, even in cases where penicillin and sulfa drugs did not work. Stinging nettle activates the body and benefits a weak heart, reduces blood pressure in arteriosclerosis, soothes the nerves and stops nosebleeds.[39]

In order to strengthen the hair, massage the scalp every day with stinging nettle vinegar. This vinegar is prepared by boiling 200 grams of stinging nettle in one liter of water and one-half liter ordinary vinegar. This mixture should simmer for thirty minutes. Strain it and preserve the liquid. It helps, as well, in cleansing the circulation, reactivating the body, and stopping internal gastrointestinal bleeding, hemorrhoids, arteriosclerosis, hypertension and digestive disorders. These diseases are treated by eating the soft parts of the nettle with salad or by drinking 100-125 grams of stinging nettle juice.

Boil one teaspoon of stinging nettle in one-half cup of water for ten minutes. This remedy is an effective treatment for renal colic due to the fact that it also helps produce urine, which results in the prevention of this disease.

---

[39] To stop a nosebleed, to do so, dip a piece of cotton in stinging nettle juice and block the nostril with it.

Wheat

In Arabic, wheat has many names. It is one of the most ancient foods humanity has ever known. Therefore, it had a very high status in ancient medicine.

Wheat contains many minerals, such as potassium, sodium, magnesium, phosphorus, iron, calcium, silicone, sulfur, as well as starch, glucose, cellulose and vitamins A and B.

Wheat has great importance in nutrition and medicine. Therefore, black bread, which consists of whole wheat, is considered a truly beneficial and most nutritious food. White bread is empty of the bran that contains most of the nutrients, vitamins and minerals. Wheat's calcium helps build of bones, its silicone helps strengthen hair, its iodine balances glandular function and relaxes and soothes the body. Its potassium, sodium and magnesium build body tissue and digestive liquids. Wheat is prescribed for the treatment of the conditions listed below.

Boil a handful of wheat bran in one liter of water and then drink the water. It soothes coughs, mild colds, chronic diarrhea and fever. If you add honey to this mixture, it will help treat gastric ulcers and constipation.

Washing the face frequently with boiled bran water both beautifies and cleanses the face from freckles. To treat sprains, prepare a poultice made of bran mixed with vinegar. For the treatment of rheumatism, prepare a bath by boiling one kilogram of bran in five liters of water for thirty minutes and then add this concentrated mixture to the tub.

For the treatment of dermatitis and other skin disorders, mix some wheat flour in some warm water and then smear it on the infected areas. Tie a bandage to hold the dough in place until morning. The infection, swelling and pain will be over, inshā'a-llāh (﷾).

Bread is an important and indispensable food for human beings. One way to absorb all of its benefits is to chew your bread longer. Dried bread is digested more easily; therefore, it is better to toast bread before eating it.

It is easy to get the beneficial nutrients of the bran—simply add one gram of bran powder to your food. It is better if it is added to foods that are not well-digested or do not provide enough nutritional value. Such a small amount of bran gives tremendous benefit in cases of indigestion and intestinal colic. Both adults and children can take it, and at the same time, it is considered a spice that adds a pleasant flavor.

Scientifically, it has been proven that eating whole wheat bread strengthens the nervous system, the brain, reproductive organs, circulation, the skeleton, teeth and hair. It adjusts thyroid function, stimulates the digestive juices, protects the immune system and provides vitality and activity.

Dr. Fania described wheat as a botanical egg, for it consists of many active ingredients and essential nutrients.

Coffee

The history of coffee goes far back into the past. It was said that an Arab was herding his sheep until suddenly the sheep began to act strangely. They became extremely active. He watched them closely until he noticed that they were eating fruit from a certain tree. So he, too, decided to give it a try and after eating it he felt incredibly vital and energetic. So the shepherd began to spread this story to the villagers and this fruit became very popular.

It has also been named "the wine of the righteous" because groups of Sufis tend to drink coffee in order to stay awake for reading and learning.

The coffee tree is an evergreen and it grows to be about three meters high. It should always be trimmed in order to maintain a certain height. This tree blooms for the first time after it becomes three to four years old. The coffee fruit has two beans inside of it and it is egg-shaped. In the beginning, the coffee fruit is dark green and after six months when it is ripe, it becomes yellow and then it turns crimson.

At that stage, the coffee beans are picked and preserved in large, sealed containers. Then they are soaked in water for twenty-four hours until they ferment and the sticky substances dissolve. For four days they are washed and dried in the sun and afterward, the beans are roasted to sharpen their special flavor and refreshing smell. The roasting takes place in special machines with metal cylinders in order to dry the beans as much as possible. The sugar in the coffee beans is caramelized, its acids are formed and its caffeine is increased and concentrated.

A substance called caffeoyl is one of the most important materials found in the beans, for it is responsible for coffee's special smell.

Coffee beans contain 10-13% protein, 15% carbohydrates and 10-13% dextrin.[40]

Caffeine is the most active ingredient in the coffee bean. Tannins come second; therefore, it is better to boil coffee properly in order to prevent constipation. Coffee's effect varies from one person to another. Some people are allergic to coffee.

Coffee has an activating and stimulating influence on the central nervous system, especially the cerebral cortex, for it speeds up the heart rate.

Coffee is also used to fight the effects of some drugs (i.e. opium); such symptoms are drowsiness and a heavy effect on the nervous system. It also has a slight impact on urine production and thus, unroasted beans are used to treat diarrhea and some cases of fever.

A normal adult can drink about one-half cup of coffee daily without being influenced by it. However, it is prohibited for children. Adults can consume coffee in small amounts, for it is considered healthy to do so. After drinking one-quarter cup of coffee there is a calm feeling that can last for several hours, which is the influence of the caffeine. Drinking one-quarter cup of coffee after meals helps digestion. Drinking coffee on an empty stomach is extremely dangerous.

If coffee is consumed excessively, it becomes toxic because it stimulates the nervous system which can lead to permanent agitation, chronic poisoning, digestive disorders and it can change the color of the complexion. Coffee is absolutely forbidden for children, people suffering from nervous system disorders, people with heart disease and hypertension.

---

[40] Fatty substances which are formed from oleic and palmitic acids.

Flax (Common Flax or Linseed)

Flax is always planted in Egypt and it is very popular. Its seeds are used after they ripen to treat infection and pain, for they contain essential oils and laxative, analgesic gel-like substances.

In ancient medicine, treatments with flax seed were very popular. Many medical scholars have spoken of flax and one of them is Dāwūd Al-Anṭākī (﷽) who mentioned in *The Memento*, "Crush and grind flax seed with hot water and wax. Place it on tumors and they will soon be healed, chronic headaches will be reduced, the face will get younger and the skin and hair will become healthier. When it is drunk, it cures lung, liver and the spleen infections. It helps clean the intestines from all old feces and it enhances the production of semen. According to many people's experiences, adding flax seed to honey and pepper increases sexual desire and performance. However, this remedy leads to poor eyesight—which can be fixed with coriander—and it weakens the digestion temporarily—which can be fixed with a mixture of honey and vinegar. If both disorders occur, then take honey between three and ten times a day or drink fenugreek tea."

Boil some flax seed and add the liquid to the bathtub or use it in an enema to help soothe, relax and alleviate infected areas, ulcers or blisters. This treatment has been known to heal the urinary tract and to facilitate the secretion of urine, especially in cases of urinary tract diseases and blood in the urine.

Prepare a flax seed poultice by boiling the seeds in water and then soak the poultice in the liquid. Place the poultice on the painful ulcers or infected tumors. This poultice should be used while hot and all hair should be removed from the areas to be treated.

In modern medicine, flax seed is prescribed for some medical conditions. Some of these diseases are mentioned by Dr. Amīn Ruwīhā in his book *Herbal Medicine*; we will summarize it as follows.

Use a hot poultice of flax seed for treating gastrointestinal colic and infections, parotitis,[41] lymph node adenitis (infection), abscesses, solid ulcers and skin diseases that involve draining pus or skin flaking. The poultice is prepared by mixing powdered flax in hot water until the mixture becomes a paste. Smear the paste onto two pieces of gauze and then place the poultice on the infected areas. Then cover the whole thing with another piece of wool. For burns, mix flax oil with egg whites and apply the mixture to the burn.

From Inside

Flax seed contains an essential oil and a type of gel that is soothing to the mucosal membranes of the skin. This substance also acts as an analgesic for respiratory system pain and disorders accompanied by a dry cough. Such painful coughs come especially after the measles, and flax seed puts an end to them. As for the digestive system, flax seed prevents constipation, especially when accompanied by painful cramps.

Flax seed also eases gastrointestinal colic, the abdominal pain associated with gallbladder or kidney stones, as well as urinary tract pain. In any of these cases, drink one-quarter to one-half cup of a flax seed and water mixture; drink it in little sips. The mixture is prepared by adding one teaspoon of flax seed to one-quarter liter of water and boiling it for three minutes. Then let the mixture steep for ten minutes.

However, this mixture does not really help in the treatment of constipation; therefore, for constipation it is preferable to add one to two teaspoons of flax seed to warm water and mix it (without boiling) and then drink it down all at once. It is also possible to simply eat one teaspoon of whole flax seed (not ground). Chew the flax and then swallow it with a little water in the morning and at night. To improve

---

[41] An inflammation of one or both parotid glands.

the taste of flax seed, mix 1 teaspoon of flax seed with 1 teaspoon of honey.

Flax seed oil is also used to treat the pain associated with kidney stones and it can help dissolve or remove them if they are small. In this case, take four teaspoons of flax seed oil daily in small doses.

Intestinal ulcers are also treated with flax seed oil by taking three teaspoons of it once a day.

Cabbage

Cabbage is considered one of the ancient plants; it has a prolonged history and many stories associated with it.

In ancient medicine, Shaykh Ibn Sīnā (ﷺ) mentions in his book al-Qānūn that there are tremendous benefits from eating cabbage. This plant is most beneficial in the treatment of Parkinson's disease and gout[42] and arthritic pain.[43] When cabbage is mixed with fenugreek powder and used as a bandage, it heals both arthritic pain and gout.

It was also said by the Greek physician, pharmacologist and botanist, Pedanius Dioscorides, that consuming cabbage heals visual impairments, clears the voice and repairs vocal cord disorders,[44] however, it may cause some gastric disorders. Cabbage juice helps treat spleen disorders and jaundice, diuresis, menstrual pain and gastrointestinal worms or parasites.[45]

In modern medicine, cabbage comes in many colors and shapes. If it is cooked properly and prepared suitably, then it is considered a most valuable and nutritious foods, in addition to its medical usages. It is also considered one of the most loved and delicious foods in traditional Arab cooking. It provides the body with considerable amounts of iron and therefore, it is considered one of the most important foods for the blood. Cabbage consists of a high percentage of water, reaching about 92%. Some of the most important medical features of cabbages are:

- Cabbage sterilizes and strengthens body tissue, which in return heals wounds and enhances the human body's natural defenses.

---

[42] If taken with fenugreek.
[43] When cooked and placed on the infected joints.
[44] Treat vocal cord disorders by chewing cabbage and sucking its juice.
[45] By adding it to lupin juice.

- Cabbage eases the metabolism when digesting carbohydrates and it creates a suitable atmosphere for the cells to be able to absorb oxygen naturally.

- Given the fact that it is rich in chlorophyll, it increases the hemoglobin in the body. It also has a high percentage of vitamins A and C and more; it is rich in phosphorus, calcium, iron, arsenic, copper, iodine and sodium.

- Additionally, it is one of the foods able to reduce blood sugar levels, making it a good food for diabetics.

Scientists find that it is most vital to consume cabbage when it is fresh; when cabbage is fresh it provides the body with the mental and physical energy to naturally maintain daily functioning, it makes the body stronger against many elements of fatigue and stress, it enhances the immune system and the body's and natural defenses, and it helps in cases of general weakness and premature aging. They add that cabbage juice is a great treatment for anemia resulting from respiratory system disorders, digestive disorders (i.e. cramps, gastrointestinal ulcers and parasites), reproductive system diseases and urinary tract diseases (i.e. bladder stones and urolithiasis).

Coriander

Coriander was well-known in ancient medicine. Some ancient physicians mentioned that coriander juice mixed with vinegar and flower oil helps infected skin tumors. Gargling with its juice helps heal mouth and tongue ulcers and removes onion and garlic odors. Its juice benefits the eyes, strengthens the stomach and stops diarrhea. Its juice also prevents thirst, heartburn, itchiness, scabies[46] and satiation.[47] It strengthens the heart and prevents palpitations,[48] prevents hallucinations, soothes headaches[49] and reduces the desire for high sugar consumption.

In modern medicine, coriander is described as a strengthening digestive stimulant. It expels gases, it is antispasmodic and calms headaches, and it benefits the treatment of hypertension and arteriosclerosis. Coriander contains a good amount of iodine, which slows the absorption of alcohol in the body; this is why people who drink alcoholic beverages eat roasted coriander before drinking in an attempt to hide the effects of intoxication.

Balsamic oil is extracted from coriander, which also contains a type of alcohol called banalol. Therefore, these features explain how coriander is able to treat the following conditions.

For indigestion: soak twenty to thirty grams of coriander leaves in one liter of water. Strain it and drink the liquid in order to heal indigestion.

For bad breath: crush fifty grams of coriander leaves with forty grams of sugar cane. Mix and take one teaspoon one hour after meals with a little water.

---

[46] Eat the herb and apply its juice to the skin.
[47] Drink coriander juice with some sugar.
[48] Eat dried coriander.
[49] Drink coriander juice with thyme and sugar.

Cumin

In ancient medicine, many physicians spoke of cumin's benefits, some of which are: it generates urine, expels gases, benefits abdominal cramps and bloating.[50] Cumin stops the uterus from constantly secreting liquids, helps epistaxis,[51] benefits liver function,[52] prevents drooling,[53] calms hiccups,[54] eliminates gastrointestinal worms and parasites, brightens the face,[55] benefits the treatment of painful urination and urinary retention, and stops toothaches and colds.[56]

In modern medicine, cumin is described as an effective way to increase appetite. It fights spasticity, generates breast milk and helps digestion. It has most of the anise plant features and advantages. However, it irritates the mucus membranes and, therefore, should not be excessively consumed. Using its powder helps resolve some cases of deafness and disorders of the ear. In cases of breast inflammation and testicle inflammation, place poultices prepared with cumin powder on the infected areas.

For Spasticity and Gastric Gases

1. Add 1 teaspoon of cumin to 1 liter water and boil.

2. Drink ¼ cup of the mixture 30 minutes before meals, 3 times a day for 15 days in a row.

For Breastfeeding Mothers

- Add 1 gram of cumin powder to some honey and eat.

---

[50] Nosebleed. Cook in oil, mix with barley and then use as an enema.
[51] For severe nose bleeds, place cumin powder close to the nose and inhale it.
[52] Mix with vinegar.
[53] Chew with vinegar and swallow.
[54] Drink cumin with vinegar.
[55] Boil cumin, cool and then wash with the mixture.
[56] Cook cumin with thyme, cool, and drink and gargle it.

White Turnip

In the past, people used to eat turnips roasted with potatoes. It was said that the Greek physician Pedanius Dioscorides ordered his patients to bathe in turnip juice. It was also said in ancient times that midwives used to place poultices made of turnip on a breastfeeding women's breasts if they became swollen, inflamed, or if they needed to produce more milk.

As for the rest of turnip's advantages as told by the ancients, Dāwūd Al-Anṭākī (⌘) said that turnips cleanse the body of waste—even the urine. They clear blockages from the vessels and help heal coughs. Turnip seeds enhance sexual desire and dissolve gallstones. Crushing turnip roots and placing them on skin tumors will help them to quickly heal and disappear. Applying turnip juice to the face removes freckles. Eating and applying turnip oil to the skin helps eliminate fatigue and gastrointestinal gas. However, turnips generate gas, but this can be treated by drinking a mixture of vinegar and honey.

In modern medicine, turnip is described as an energizer, sterilizer, generator of urine, moisturizer, lung cleanser, laxative, remover of fatigue, dissolver of gallstones, cough and cold fighter and an anti-obesity food. For the treatment of the above-mentioned cases, soak turnips in water or milk and then drink the liquid. For every one hundred grams of turnip, add one liter water or milk.

For Gallstones
1. Boil 6 grams of turnip seeds with some linden flowers.
2. Strain and drink.

- This also benefits coughs and cold diseases.

Eating fresh turnips (straight from the ground without cooking them) heals many cases of adolescent acne and eczema. Gargling with turnip water heals diphtheria; this is prepared by chopping one big turnip and boiling it in one-half liter of water for several minutes. Strain and then gargle the liquid.

Cracking Skin Due to Exposure to Cold

1. Cook 1 turnip with its peel.

2. Remove it as it softens and slice it into 2 halves.

3. Take one half and rub the cracked areas with it. Then squeeze it so that some turnip juice drips on the affected areas.

- This treatment can be also applied to abscesses or skin cysts.

Because turnips are difficult to digest, they are not recommended for people who suffer from a weak stomach or intestines. Healthy people can consume as much as possible, but you must make sure they are very fresh—otherwise, they will be very hard to digest.

Eating cooked turnip is recommended in order to prevent them from causing gastric gas. Obese people should not eat them. Also, people at risk for skin diseases should not eat them, for they are rich in sulfur. Turnips are completely prohibited for diabetics and kidney patients.

Lemon

The lemon tree is one of the oldest trees people have ever known. The Egyptians used lemons to treat many diseases, especially poisoning. They used to call the lemon tree "benzhir," which is a Persian word meaning anti-toxin.

Dāwūd Al-Anṭākī (☙) mentioned lemon's advantages in the treatment of heartburn, headaches, thirst, vomiting, nausea, food poisoning and most types of toxicity. Lemons stimulate the appetite, balance your consumption of foods, prevent food poisoning and fight many toxins. Its peel is most effective in the treatment of poisoning and toxicity. Its seeds also have a great effect in healing disease. It was said that lemon is as good as citron. In the past, citron was given the name "the Persian apple" for its tremendous medicinal benefits. The thinner the lemon peel, the more effective it becomes for colic and gas.

Dry some lemons, crush them, mix in an equal amount of sugar, and then eat them. This remedy will remove headaches, dizziness and it opens blocked arteries. Lemon juice clears the face of freckles, vitiligo and itchiness. Making a paste out of its leaves, flower petals and peels results in a wonderful remedy that is better than vinegar for patients. Adding some salt to the previous mixture strengthens the stomach and removes any waste products. If lemon is sniffed and smelled, it easily puts an end to a runny nose and a stuffy chest.

In modern medicine, lemon is considered to be one of the fruits richest in vitamin C, which prevents scurvy and its symptoms like headache, general weakness, indigestion, dental erosion, skin spots, bleeding and enlargement of the limbs and joints.

One hundred grams of lemon juice consists of fifty micrograms of vitamin C,[57] eighty micrograms of niacin[58] and forty micrograms of riboflavin.[59]

Lemon also contains a high percentage of citrine, which strengthens the walls of the blood vessels.

There are many nutrients found in the lemon; the lemon contains 8.3% carbohydrates and minerals such as calcium, potassium and iron, which help maintain the proper alkalinity of the body.

Lemon juice is used in the treatment of mouth rash and tongue infections by rubbing lemon juice on the infected surfaces. Ancient Egyptians used it to strengthen the gums and to eliminate mouth microbes, which cause moldiness in the mouth. Gargling with its juice helps cure sore throat and other throat infections.[60] Adding 2% potassium chlorate and 1% lemon brine (lemon-salt solution) to drinking water protects the drinker from cholera.

Lemon juice also has helps in the treatment of gout, which was called "the king's malady," by dissolving the condensed salts in the joints. Therefore, it is also treats rheumatism. Use lemon to treat headaches and sunstrokes by placing a poultice of lemon juice on the forehead.

Lemon activates the kidneys and the liver and it is one of the most important sources of vitamin C. The human body cannot store vitamin C in the body so it must regularly receive it from food.

Lemon peel has a beautiful odor and for this reason, it is used in perfume. In addition, it is very effective in expelling gastrointestinal gas. Lemon oil is a beneficial medicine for eliminating gastrointestinal

---

[57] Which prevents nervous system inflammation.
[58] Vitamin B_3, known as essential to the prevention of pellagra.
[59] Vitamin B_2, which is needed for the oxidation, metabolism and normal growth of the body.
[60] Dilute with some water before gargling.

parasites and worms. Lemon seeds are quite bitter, thus, they are detoxifying; they cleanse the digestive system of waste and parasites and they are used to strengthen medications and powders.

Generally, lemon activates the muscles and fights fatigue and cold. Many experiments were done with small animals by giving them some lemon to eat. Those that consumed the lemon benefited from its vitamin C and had a stronger resistance to extreme cold compared to those that did not eat lemon. Therefore, lemon became a great remedy against winter sicknesses, for it enhances the body's resistance, protects kidney cells and eliminates germs, especially the kind of germs that attack the thyroid gland.

Lemon is prescribed for all people of all ages without exception. Lemon juice should be diluted with water in certain cases.

Unfortunately, lemon can sometimes cause harm, for it has a relatively high concentration of citric and malic acids, which can sometimes cause digestive tract bleeding, gastrointestinal ulcers and damage to tooth enamel.

However, drinking lemon juice diluted with some water on an empty stomach every morning is very beneficial. It cleanses the stomach from waste and toxins, protects the liver and body cells and reinforces the immune system resistance. When several drops of lemon juice are added to cow's milk, it provides some of the basic nutrition a child needs.

There are additional popular recipes using lemon for the treatment of disease, as follows:

To Expel Intestinal Worms and Parasites

1. Soak 1 whole, crushed lemon in water for 2 hours.

2. Squeeze all parts well before removing the lemon from the mixture, and then strain.

3. Add some honey to the lemon liquid and drink it before bedtime. This can be repeated as required.

Liver Infections

1. Slice 3 lemons and soak them in hot water in the evening.

2. Let it sit until morning and then drink the water on an empty stomach.

Obesity

1. Soak some cumin in hot water. Add a sliced lemon and let it sit all night.

2. Drink it in the morning on an empty stomach.

Abdominal Swelling

1. Add 5-10 drops of lemon juice to some honey.

2. Take in several doses.

To Purify the Blood

- Drink about 100 grams of lemon juice daily.

To Stop a Nosebleed

- Block the bleeding nostril with a piece of cotton soaked in lemon juice.

Constipation

1. Boil 1 lemon in water for 10 minutes.

2. When the lemon peel becomes softer, slice it in half and squeeze the juice into a cup.

3. Add 2 teaspoons of glycerin to the lemon juice and fill the rest of the cup with honey.

4. Mix well and drink.

Inflammation of the Trachea and Nighttime Attacks of Coughing

- Take 1 teaspoon of the previously mentioned constipation remedy above before bedtime and during the night.

Chronic Cough

1. Take 1 teaspoon of the previously mentioned constipation remedy in the morning immediately after waking up, another before noon, a third in the afternoon, a fourth before dinner and a fifth before bedtime.

2. These dosages can be reduced as you improve.

Lemon as a Cosmetic

Blackheads

1. Wash the face with hot water in the evening and then apply a mixture of equal parts glycerin, alcohol and lemon juice to the face.

2. In the morning, wash the face again with hot water and then rub the blackheads with a piece of cotton.

3. Repeat this procedure for a week.

Facial Cleanser (Especially for Large Pores)

- Use lemon juice to clean the face daily, for it benefits the skin and tightens its tissue. Oily skin gets dirty faster than other types—however, lemon helps prevent this.

Nutrient-Rich Facial Mask

1. Mix the juice of 1 lemon with 1 beaten egg white.

2. Wash and dry your face properly.

3. Apply the mixture to the face and around the eyes (but not too close to the eyes).

4. Leave this mask for 15 minutes until it dries.

5. Wash with warm water, using a piece of cotton.

Scalp Treatment

Lemon juice is also very beneficial for the hair and scalp.

- Massage the scalp with lemon juice and then wash with warm water.

Wounds

- Lemon is an astringent substance that helps shrink the blood vessels. Therefore, it is very effective in helping wounds to heal more quickly when used on bandages.

Peppermint

Peppermint is considered a medicinal herb. The first Arab physicians discussed its benefits frequently. Dāwūd Al-Anṭākī (☀) said that peppermint prevents nausea and hiccups. When it is taken with honey and vinegar, it is the best cure for gastrointestinal parasites. Also, it prevents satiety and the formation of gastric acidity. If it is chewed, it can soothe toothaches and strengthen the heart. It is preferable to dry peppermint in the shade in order to preserve its benefits and refreshing smell.

In modern medicine, it is said that peppermint contains an essential oil called menthol and some menthon, in addition to tannins which prevent cramps and cure infections.

Peppermint is described as the "heart's friend," and it is also the friend of the nervous and digestive systems. It strengthens the body, calms the nerves, comforts the intestines from gas, enhances the performance of the liver and spleen, benefits the treatment of cough and asthma, facilitates breathing, generates urine, reduces the sensitivity of gastric mucus membranes and is used topically as a treatment for rheumatism, arthritis and infection.

Gargling with peppermint water heals the gums and teeth while providing a pleasant odor to the mouth. Due to the fact it contains menthol, it expels germs and insects that carry germs.

In order to treat mastitis, prepare a poultice with peppermint leaves, vinegar and the inner part of white bread. Mix the ingredients together and put them in a cloth to be placed on the infected breast.

The essential oil of peppermint is used to massage areas infected with rheumatism. This soothes the pain and heals the infection.

Taken internally: a peppermint emulsion is one of the best remedies for treating gallbladder disorders, intestinal colic, menstrual pain and gastrointestinal disorders. This emulsion provides the body with activity and vitality.

Prepare this emulsion by adding one teaspoon of peppermint leaves to a quarter cup of hot water. Drink one-half to three-quarters of a cup daily; it can be mixed with milk, if desired.

Also, peppermint enhances sexual desire. Make this remedy by adding five grams of peppermint leaves to a quarter cup of water. If desired, one can add some hawthorn fruit in order to strengthen its effect. It is advised to avoid drinking this emulsion when there is fever and vomiting, for it will stimulate vomiting, dry up the mouth and create a strong thirst.

Al-Hijama

(Bleeding Cupping)

This is an alternative medicine that heals many diseases. It is said that the Prophet Muḥammad (ﷺ), may the peace and blessings of Allāh (ﷻ) be upon him said, "Healing is by 3 (means): a drink of honey, cupping and cauterizing with fire; however, I forbid my nation to use cauterization." (Bukhārī 7:585)

Cupping is performed by making a tiny incision in the skin with a sharp blade. The cups then are placed on the incised area. Due to the cups' reduced air pressure, a suction of the skin is created and the blood begins to be drawn into the cups.

Additionally, the virtue of cupping is clarified in the Prophet's saying (ﷺ), peace and blessings of Allāh (ﷻ) upon him, "The best of remedies is al-ḥijāma." Al-ḥijāma has many benefits: it purifies the body's surface and it heals shoulder pain, sore throat, toothache, nose and eye disorders, headache and forgetfulness.

Ibn Mājah (ؓ) describes the best times to perform this treatment, "Al-ḥijāma is most healing on the seventeenth, nineteenth and twenty-first days of the (lunar) month. It heals every disease except poisoning. It is most disliked when one is full (when one has eaten recently); it is most effective when one is hungry."

Imām Aḥmad bin Ḥanbal (ؓ) was asked which days were most dangerous to perform al-ḥijāma. He answered, "Wednesdays and Saturdays." The Prophet Muḥammad (ﷺ), may the peace and blessings of Allāh (ﷻ) be upon him, used to receive al-ḥijāma while he was fasting. He used to have al-ḥijāma performed on the ridge between the shoulder blades and on the two veins on both sides of the neck (the carotid arteries).[61] Also, al-ḥijāma was done on the back of his neck and the back of his foot. It can be performed on any area of the body that is ill.

It was said that the Prophet Muḥammad (ﷺ) used al-ḥijāma on many places of his body, as mentioned by Ibn al-Qayyim (ﷺ) in his book *Zād al-mi'ād*. He mentioned that using bleeding cupping on the area between the shoulder blades benefits the treatment of shoulder pain. Receiving al-ḥijāma on the vein on both sides of the neck helps headaches and head pains (toothache, ear pain, eye pain, nose pain and throat pain) which occur as a result of excessive blood, toxic blood, or both.

Al-ḥijāma is also frequently used to discharge magic and shayṭānic possession. One of the most effective benefits of al-ḥijāma is its ability to expel a custodian of magic from the body. The custodian of magic is the jinn entrusted with the magic. It is known, as mentioned in the prophetic sayings, that Iblīs moves in the human body with the blood as it circulates. The jinn also live in the circulation and there they cast magic. If the evil substance is removed from the blood, the bewitched person is healed, inshā'a-llāh (ﷺ). This should also be accompanied by Qur'ānic recitation, specifically the verses that stop magical influences and the protective ruqyā which are āyātu-l-kursī, sūratu-l-ikhlās, sūratu-l-falaq and sūratu-n-nās.

Bleeding cupping also helps when the human body is possessed by shayṭān. In this case, while performing cupping recite the verses of protection: sūratu-l-ikhlās 3 times, sūratu-l-falaq 3 times and then sūratu-n-nās 3 times. One of the signs that the treatment has succeeded is abundant blood flow from the incisions into the cups. Usually, the kind of blood that comes out in such cases is dried, crusted blood that is not very liquid. This treatment should be repeated until the person is totally healed, inshā'a-llāh (ﷺ).

---

[61] Shaykh Muhammad Sa'id al-Jamal ar-Rifa'i ash-Shadhuli, *The Medicine of the Prophet*. Petaluma: Sidi Muhammad Press, 2006. p. 85.

As already mentioned, the sign that a jinn has been expelled from the body is the removal of a considerably large amount of crusted blood that is not liquid.

When Using al-Hijama to Expel a Jinn

1. One should use al-ḥijāma to expel the jinn first from the blood by reciting the appropriate verses for discharging magic and invoking protection on any part of the body (the last five āyāt of sūratu-l-ḥashr). If the crusted blood does not emerge after this recitation, the patient should be sure to do all of his/her ṣalāh, make dhikr and recite sūratu-l-baqara (or listen to it daily).

2. After the treatment the patient should wash his body with Qur'ānic water[62] and drink some of it, too. Do this for 2-4 weeks.

3. Next, the patient should repeat, "lā 'ilāha 'illa-llāh" without stopping until a tingling feeling is sensed at the tips of the fingers. Al-ḥijāma can be performed on the hand if the tingling sensation does not stop, which means that the jinn has not left the body yet.

Al-ḥijāma can also be performed on the back of the patient between the shoulders. It is extremely important that the person who performs al-ḥijāma be experienced in order for the treatment to succeed. The patient should wash his body with Qur'ānic water prior to the treatment, in addition to perfuming the body with non-alcoholic perfumes, such as musk and pure saffron. This mixture of water and odors must be applied to the body until 1 week after the winter season ends.

Know my brothers and sisters, al-ḥijāma grants great healing from many diseases by Allāh taʿālā's will (﷾). However, one should remember that the remedy will be prescribed only after a

---

[62] Water over which verses from the Qur'ān have been recited.

knowledgeable diagnosis. If, and only if, the remedy agrees with the illness, Allāh ta'ālā (ﷻ) grants the healing if He wills.

According to the visible secrets of al-ḥijāma that were witnessed by many people, for anyone who suffers from headaches or pain in certain places and has al-ḥijāma performed in both the right place and the right time, Allāh ta'ālā (ﷻ) grants the healing. This is from Allāh's abundant giving.

As for its hidden secrets, al-ḥijāma is not just for physical pain. Its effects go deeper because it is the sunna. So follow what the Prophet (ﷺ) said and receive al-ḥijāma in the way that he taught us.

The Placement of al-Hijama and its Relationship to Disease

- **To benefit the shoulders and throat** place al-ḥijāma on the back of the neck between the shoulder blades.
- **To benefit all parts of the head** (headaches, eyes, mouth, nose, ears and teeth), place al-ḥijāma on both sides of the neck on the veins.
- **To benefit toothaches, face problems and faces, as well as healing speech difficulties resulting from tongue disorders,** place al-ḥijāma beneath the chin.
- **To benefit foot pain**, place al-ḥijāma on the back of the foot.
- **To benefit joint pain**, place al-ḥijāma above the ankles (above the protruding bones).
- **To prevent swelling of the knee joints and rheumatic diseases** in those areas, place al-ḥijāma on both sides of the knees.
- **To benefit headaches and shoulder pain**, place al-ḥijāma on the back of the neck.

- To **heal shortness of breath and backache**, place al-ḥijāma at the center of the back under the shoulder blades.

- To **benefit back pain, stiffness of the legs and impotence**, place al-ḥijāma at the bottom of the back on both sides of the spine.

- To **heal headaches, dizziness and eye pain**, place al-ḥijāma on the forehead, making a very small incision and using a small cup.

- To **heal migraines** (chronic and periodic), place al-ḥijāma on both sides of the top of the head.

- On any place of the body that there is either **an older jinn or a baby jinn and they are not able to gather themselves in one specific spot to get out**, place al-ḥijāma on one certain place and recite the verses of gathering and expelling—the last 5 āyāt of sūratu-l-ḥashr.

Al-ḥijāma should be avoided when someone is recovering from a debilitating illness. It should also be avoided if someone has a weak body, is menstruating, pregnant, or in nifās (post-partum time when still bleeding). Diabetics should be treated very carefully with really special people unless the diabetes is very serious.

Times for al-Hijama

There are specific times preferable for performing al-ḥijāma; one is at the beginning of the 19th day of the Islamic (lunar) month. Ancient knowledgeable people in al-ḥijāma claim that on this particular day, the circulation in the human body begins to "boil," meaning it becomes empowered. All of the waste and dirt produced during times of pain is pushed out toward the skin and the surface of the body. Therefore, bleeding cupping helps the body to easily discharge this waste in just several minutes.

Although these facts have their significance in the world of medicine, Imām al-Bukhārī (ﷺ) states otherwise about the Prophet Muḥammad (ﷺ). He said that the Prophet Muḥammad (ﷺ) received al-ḥijāma while he was on Ḥajj at the beginning of the hijri month, because he suffered from terrible headaches. This implies that al-ḥijāma can be performed at any time, but if you are in a ḥijri month, it is recommend you receive cupping at the end of the month.[63]

The way to execute al-ḥijāma is fixed and well-known to its specialists and experienced practitioners. The incision should be made—otherwise the treatment results in nothing and it might even harm the patient. At the beginning of treatment, dry cupping can be done to separate any close veins from each other.[64] When an incision is made it should be small and it should fit easily within the diameter of the cup.

People experienced in al-ḥijāma know how to apply it for different skin types and the influence skin type has on cupping. Consider sterilizing the areas before cupping with a non-alcoholic sterilizing agent. After al-ḥijāma it is recommended that the practitioner apply a mixture that is two-thirds black seed oil and one-third honey to the cuts.

---

[63] Whereas, if you are not in a ḥijri month, it is idea to receive cupping on the 19th day of the lunar month, as stated earlier.
[64] In dry cupping the cups are applied without making any incisions first.

Gynecology and Childbirth

A mixture of boiled black seed, chamomile and honey is the best remedy for facilitating childbirth.

When used as a vaginal shower, black seed provides great benefit to women. You can also use a few drops of black seed oil with every beverage to prevent gynecological disorders.

These available and easily prepared home remedies are mercy and a blessing for women so that they do not have to go to the gynecologist unless it is truly necessary.

Infertility

Black Seed, Fenugreek, Radish Seed Remedy

1. Thanks to Allāh taʿālā (ﷻ), three things are always available: ground black seed, finely ground fenugreek seeds and radish seeds. Mix these three ingredients in equal amounts to form a paste.

2. Take 1 teaspoon of this paste in the morning and 1 teaspoon at night with ½ cup of honey.

3. Follow this with a large cup of camel's milk.[65]

4. Inshā'a-llāh (ﷻ), your desire will be achieved; but if it is not, it is Allāh's will (ﷻ).

Date Palm Pollen Remedy

• Women, before sexual intercourse insert date palm pollen into the uterus and pray to be granted with righteous offspring.

---

[65] You cannot substitute a different type of milk. If you cannot acquire camel's milk in the U.S., have it shipped from elsewhere.

Bird Brains[66] and Horse Milk Remedy

- Add a mixture of bird brain and horse milk to a piece of wool, tie it properly and then insert it into the vagina as close as possible to the uterus; this speeds up the process of getting pregnant.

Rabbit Egg Fertilization Remedy

Rabbit rennet[67] is very helpful in the process of egg fertilization.

1. Take some rabbit rennet and put it in a piece of wool.

2. Insert the wool into the vagina.

3. Do this the moment you are cleansed from your menstrual period. This helps in getting pregnant.

Olive Oil and Rabbit

1. Add some olive oil to a rabbit's gallbladder and mix them together.

2. Dip a piece of cotton into the mixture and insert it as a suppository into the vagina. This will speed up the process of becoming pregnant.

Cumin and Lime Juice

- Drink a mixture of lime juice and cumin to enhance your fertility.

To Facilitate Birth and to Remove the Placenta

Thyme and Fenugreek

1. Boil thyme and fenugreek seeds together in some water.

2. Allow it to boil on low heat for several minutes.

3. Strain and drink it during labor.

---

[66] Use the brains of a flying bird (i.e., not a chicken).
[67] A complex of enzymes produced in the stomach to digest the mother's milk.

3. Fenugreek Wash and Soak

- Boil fenugreek in water and wash the vagina with the water.

- If a woman who is about to give birth sits in fenugreek water, this will ease the birth and it will help the placenta to drop easily, as well.

- Sitting in fenugreek water before the birth begins also cleanses the uterus after the birth, inshā'a-llāh (ﷻ).

Saffron and Rose Water

- Mix about 5 grams of saffron with a little water and rose water.

- This helps to speed up the labor process, according to women who have successfully used this remedy.

To Ease Labor for a Barren Woman Who Took a Long Time to Get Pregnant

- Grind together bird brains[68] with horse milk and drink.

To Accelerate Contractions and Increase Breast Milk Production

Anise tea is most efficient in accelerating labor contractions, as well as increasing milk production. To prepare this tea:

1. Add 1 teaspoon of anise seeds to ¼ cup of very hot water.

2. Strain, cool and then drink several times during labor.

Amenorrhoea[69] and Hypomenorrhoea[70]
Arugula Juice

1. Extract arugula juice by mashing its leaves and straining the juice.

---

[68] Use the brains of a flying bird (i.e., not a chicken).
[69] When a women of reproductive age isn't getting her period at all.
[70] Extremely light periods

2. Take 1 teaspoon of the juice three times a day with either water or milk. This helps generate menstrual blood.

Another way to treat this case:

• Boil 1 teaspoon of anise seeds in ¼ cup of water. Drink once a day.

Grape Leaves

1. In addition, grapes leaves are also used to treat amenorrhea caused by something other than pregnancy.

2. Soak 50 grams of grape leaves in 1 liter of cold water for several minutes.

3. Then, bring it a boil and let it simmer for ½ hour.

4. Let cool for 15 minutes. Strain the water, sweeten it with some honey and then drink ¾ cup of it after eating. This will cause the menses to flow naturally, inshā'a-llāh (🕮).

Menstrual Pain

Perhaps this is one of the most important problems women face during their menses. This pain results from the heat of the uterus as it sheds the uterine lining. To stop this pain follow these steps carefully:

Ingredients:
1 ounce raw musk
10 grams rose water
1 ounce saffron

1. Grind the saffron properly.

2. Add the rose water and then the raw musk to the saffron and grind it all together into a fine paste.

3. Add 1 liter of water and bring it to a boil on low heat.

4. Take a small piece of wood and wrap one of its ends with a piece of cloth. Dip the wood covered in cloth in the mixture and insert it into the vagina.

Another remedy for menstrual pain

Ingredients:
1 ounce saffron
5 grams rose water
1 pound honey
1 ounce amber oil
1 ounce sugar cane.

1. Grind the sugar finely with the saffron.

2. Mix in the amber oil and gradually add the rose water.

3. Finally, mix in the honey.

4. Cook on low heat until all ingredients have combined.

5. Take 1 teaspoon of this every morning and apply it as an ointment to the vagina.

6. This should be used for three weeks after your menstrual bleeding has finished.

- A woman should take into account that hot and spicy foods, such as ginger and cinnamon, are not allowed during this treatment.

- It is preferable to repeat this treatment every 1-2 menstrual cycles, for it totally eliminates menstrual pain. This is beneficial when successfully implemented and it will give you satisfactory results, inshā'a-llāh.

Impotence and Sexual Dysfunction

Sexual intercourse is a basic human need and it is just as important as any other life necessity. For many, sex is a symbol of manhood and strength; sometimes it even symbolizes dignity and the future. A man, for instance, minds less if his hair turns completely white or his skin is wrinkled than he minds learning that his sexual abilities are weakening and decreasing. This issue has overwhelmed many people and possessed their lives, both in the past and today.

Many people do not realize that there is a great difference between sexual impotence and infertility. Many physicians claim they can heal infertility; this is inaccurate if they are healing impotence, whether male or female. A woman can be at her highest level of fertility, have a regular menstrual cycle and be married to the most fertile man who produces the most sperm, but she may not get pregnant. Why? Because Allāh (ﷻ) does not wish to grant it to them yet. This is also true for infertility. No human being on earth can heal this disease for many reasons, one of which is the most important: that it does not have a cure. Healthy couples do not have children because it is Allāh's will (ﷻ), for Allāh ta'ālā (ﷻ) says:

لله ملك السماوات والأرض يخلق ما يشاء يهب لمن يشاء إناثا
ويهب لمن يشاء الذكور أو يزوجهم ذكرانا وإناثا ويجعل من
يشاء عقيما إنه عليم قدير

"Allāh (ﷻ) has control of the heavens and the earth; He creates whatever He wills.
He grants female offspring to whomever He wills, male to whomever He wills,
or both male and female and He makes whomever He wills barren:
He is the All-Knowing and the All-Powerful." (42:49-50)

These verses are a clear statement that infertility depends upon Allāh's will (ﷻ). If He wills, He grants fertility and if He wills, He prevents fertility.

Three Types of Sexual Dysfunctions and Impotence:

1. ### Lack of Semen

   This kind of weakness usually occurs because the body "lacks heat," meaning that the food consumed does not supply the body with the necessary ingredients to produce semen, like fruit (grapes and sweet fruits are the most important). However, if the condition does not improve, then the body requires a strong stimulant. However, a man should keep in mind not to have excessive sex after the treatment. The ingredients are:

   1 ounce of raw amber oil
   three leaves of sugar cane
   2 pounds of honey
   ½ cup of cow's milk (whole 4% milk)

   1. Grind the sugar cane into a powder.

   2. Heat the honey on low heat. It is best if you heat it in a bowl of hot water.

   3. In a separate saucepan, bring the milk to a boil. Pour it gradually into the honey, stirring constantly.

   4. Finally, add the amber oil and the ground sugar cane.

   5. Mix for 5-10 minutes until all ingredients are well-combined.

   6. Take 1 teaspoon of the mixture in the morning before breakfast, another before lunch and another 2 hours before bedtime.

   7. This should be repeated for three weeks, during which time the husband should decrease the amount of sexual intercourse he has with his wife. Also, he should consume an above-average amount of fruit and inshā'a-llāh (※) he will be cured.

2. **Oligospermia** is the condition of having semen with a low concentration of sperm. This condition is caused by a lack moisture in the testicles. Moisturizing elements support sperm production and they diminish when a man reduces his intake of the substances that provide this moisture. By preparing this remedy, a man can gain back this kind of moisture. The ingredients are:

½ ounce rue
½ ounce garden cress (Lepidium sativum)
3 ounces amber oil
2 ounces sugar cane
1 cup goat's milk
½ kilogram honey

1. Grind both the rue and the garden cress together and blend them with the amber oil.

2. Bring the goat's milk to a low boil.

3. As the dough is ready, slice it into 14 equal pieces.

4. Add 1 piece of the dough into 1 cup of goat's milk and add 1-2 teaspoons of honey.

5. Drink the mixture at least 2 hours before bedtime.

6. Continue this treatment for 2 continuous weeks, during which time the husband should decrease the amount of sexual intercourse he has with his wife in order to leave time for the sperm to be fully produced, inshā'a-llāh (ﷻ).

3. **Erectile Dysfunction** (ED) is due to a lack of the electrical force coming from the end of the spine. This force is required to initiate an erection. Therefore, the following concoction is very helpful in regaining this ability. The ingredients are:

2 ounces black seed

2 ounces black pepper and cinnamon
honey
½ ounce ginger
camel's milk[71]

1. Grind the black seed, black pepper and cinnamon into a fine powder.

2. Boil the camel's milk and then add 1 teaspoon of this powder and 1 teaspoon of honey to it.

3. Drink this for 2 weeks. This also is very beneficial for the brain and the electricity of the spine, which will lead to a strong erection.

Generally, the ingredients and remedies prescribed for the treatment of sexual dysfunction enhance the nervous system. As the nervous system is healed, the healing moves on to the reproductive system and, as a result it is empowered and improved.

To Increase Sexual Desire

Chickpea Water
1. Soak chickpeas in water for several hours.

2. Eat the chickpeas raw and drink the liquid with a little honey.

3. This will restore the desire for sex even after a period of depression.

Black Seed, Milk, Olive Oil, Oliban
1. Grind some black seed and add it to olive oil, milk and oliban.

2. Mix together and drink. This will remove this malady, inshā'a-llāh (ﷺ).

---

[71] You cannot substitute a different type of milk. If you cannot acquire camel's milk in the U.S., you will need to have it shipped from elsewhere.

To Enhance Sexual Performance and Reproduction

Garlic, Cloves and Milk

1. Mash some garlic cloves and cook on low heat with sheep's milk or cow's milk.

2. Add native ghee and honey.

3. This is a powerful remedy to enhance sexual performance and reproduction. Eat from this mixture frequently and you will notice the difference, inshā'a-llāh (ﷻ).

Oliban and Honey

1. Add 1 ounce of oliban to a pound of honey.

2. Heat the mixture on low heat until the oliban melts.

3. Drink on an empty stomach morning and evening while it cools.

4. Behold the wonder of this remedy in enhancing the sexual strength.

Onions and Honey

1. Juice some onions and add honey to it.

2. Boil it on low heat until the onion juice evaporates and the honey remains.

3. Put aside to cool.

4. Add 1 ounce of this onion-honey mixture to 3 ounces of water.

5. Soak with a sliced lemon for a whole day.

6. Drink the mixture before going to sleep. This remedy both enhances the erection and sexual ability.

- Also, eating egg yolk frequently on an empty stomach strengthens sexual ability. Taking egg yolks with crushed onions has an amazingly strong effect!

- Drinking camel's milk with honey frequently enhances sexual strength.[72]

- Grind celery seeds finely and add white sugar. Mix the powder with ghee made from cow butter and drink for three days.

- Add some finely ground carnation to 1 cup of milk. Drink on an empty stomach for it will enhance a man's sexual performance.

- Mix together onion juice, arugula juice, ghee and honey.

Mustard Remedy

1. Crush mustard seeds and mix them with mustard oil.

2. Apply the paste to the penis, the pubis and the area above to improve erection, as well as sexual performance.

Myrrh Remedy

1. Add 2 pieces of myrrh to about 2 teaspoons of animal fat.

2. Mix together and apply to the penis. This is a very efficient ointment to improve erection.

Egg Remedy

1. Boil 10 eggs.

2. After they are cooked, remove the yolks and put them aside to dry out completely.

3. Then put some cow's milk in a saucepan and add arugula juice to it.

4. Cook the milk, arugula juice, egg yolks and some ghee on low heat until the mixture is cooked.

5. Drink this on an empty stomach, for it improves the sexual condition.

---

[72] You cannot substitute a different type of milk. If you cannot acquire camel's milk in the U.S., you will need to have it shipped from elsewhere.

Milk, Ghee and Honey

1. In a saucepan, cook 1 pound of cow's milk, ½ pound ghee and 1 pound of honey.

2. Add to the mixture black chickpea powder (the chickpeas should have been roasted first) and stir until the mixture becomes like rock candy.

3. Take a piece of it every day and continue for three days.

4. A man should not have any sexual intercourse during the treatment until he gains back his full strength.

Chicken Gallbladder

1. Add a chicken's gallbladder to some ginger powder and ground them together into a paste.

2. Apply the paste to the penis, for it results in a delightful sexual sensation.

3. Also, adding honey to this mixture before intercourse will enhance the man's sexual performance.

The King's Paste: A Very Powerful Remedy for Reproductive Enhancement

1. Mix together 10 grams of the following herbs and seeds:

   celery seeds
   pine seeds
   ginger
   arugula seeds
   radish seeds
   tiger nut sedges (Cyperus esculentus or earth almond)
   stomach of a sandfish skink (a small lizard at the pet store)
   galangal
   walnuts
   amber oil

phrethrum (several plants of the genus Chrysanthemum)
carrot seeds
royal jelly
date palm pollen

2. As these are mixed together, add honey[73] and mix well.

3. Put the mixture in a jar to preserve it.

4. When needed, take 1 teaspoon of this mixture after lunch, for it is every man's goal.

Garlic, Cloves and Olive Oil

1. Mash some garlic cloves and fry them in olive oil until they become yellowish.

2. Preserve them in a small container.

3. Apply to the pubis by massaging the area in a circulatory motion. Leave this on for at least an hour.

4. This is a very powerful remedy to enhance sexual ability.

Black Seed, Eggs and Garlic

1. Beat 1 teaspoon of ground black seed with 7 native eggs.

2. Eat 1 teaspoon of this mixture every day and a 120 year-old man will feel like a 20 year-old, inshā'a-llāh (﷽).

3. In addition, swallow 1 clove of garlic after taking the mixture. This will help prevent high cholesterol.

4. It is recommended that a man not have a sexual intercourse when exhausted and each time before he has intercourse he should urinate and perform wuḍū' (ablution). Then, he should pray to Allāh (﷽) by saying, "Oh Allāh (﷽), distance Iblīs from me and distance him from what You have blessed me with."

---

[73] If gathering fresh honey, make sure all of the foam is removed before using it.

Onion, Honey and Black Seed

One can also prepare another remedy with similar outcome.

1. Juice three onions.

2. Strain and heat some honey until the honey's foam dissolves.

3. Place the onion juice and honey in a container and eat 1 teaspoon of it every day after every lunch.

4. It is also helpful to add black seed or radish seeds and eat it like a jam. This remedy has very powerful and immediate effects.

Honey and Onion Juice

1. Boil together 1 cup of honey and 1 cup of onion juice.

2. Let the onion juice evaporate and then take 1 teaspoon of the mixture after every meal.

- Also, one can grill onions and eat them with pistachio, palm tree pollen and honey.

Infertility (Male)

1. Extract palm date pollen and consume it immediately with 1 cup of cow's milk mixed with three milligrams of rhinoceros horn powder.[74]

2. Do this for a whole month. Inshā'a-llāh (﷾) he will be granted with offspring.

---

[74] This refers to powdered pieces of rhinoceros horn that have naturally broken off of the animal. This remedy should be only used in cases of extreme need.

To Gain Weight or for Malnutrition

Usually a person is underweight due to malnutrition, but genetics often play a role. The fact is that malnutrition does not mean lack of food consumed by a person—it means that the person does not consume a variety of foods containing certain percentages of nutrients such as minerals, carbohydrates and proteins. In addition, there are many factors other than the food he or she eats that can cause this condition, which can create psychological strain, worry and anxiety. Malnutrition can also be as a result of a poor appetite or because of certain body-system failures.

1. Crush tigernut sedges (Cyperus esculentus or earth almond) and soak them in water overnight.

2. Strain them, mash them together and then add some sugar.

3. Drink this for 12 days. This remedy will help the remediate these conditions.

The Medicinal Use of Herbs

Preserving Our Health

It has been said that the Caliph ar-Rashīd, who had a clever Christian physician, asked ʿAlī (ؓ), father of al-Ḥasan (ؓ), "Does not your book (the Qurʾān) contain anything on medicine?"

ʿAlī (ؓ) replied, "Allāh (ﷻ) has put this science in one-half of a verse in His book."

The Christian proceeded, "and what is it?"

So ʿAlī (ؓ) said, "And eat and drink but do not be extravagant." (7:31)

The Christian then asked, "And what does your prophet say about medicine?"

ʿAlī (ؓ) replied, "Our Prophet (ﷺ) has gathered this science in simple words."

He asked again, "What are they?"

So ʿAlī (ؓ) relayed the prophetic saying, "The stomach is the home of illness. A few mouthfuls of food should be enough to give a man all the strength he needs. Let one-third of your stomach for food, one-third for drink and one-third for breath."

The Christian physician said, "Your prophet did not leave anything out about medicine, even for the great Galen."[75]

It was narrated that ʿAlī ibn Abi Ṭālib (ؓ) used to say, "He who wishes to live, eat lunch like an early bird and eat dinner quickly. Eat only when your stomach is empty and drink only when you are thirsty. Do not drink a lot of water and lie down after lunch. Stroll and do not go to sleep until your bowels are emptied. Eating dried meat at night, as well as having sexual intercourse with elderly people, leads to ruin."

---

[75] A prominent physician, surgeon and philosopher.

Herbs Affecting the Jinn and Disease

Some herbs affect a human being's health and others, sometimes, lead to a human being's death. There are herbs that harm the jinn in general, and the disbelieving jinn, in particular. As illustrated, herbs are used for various medicinal purposes to maintain human health. People have used medicinal herbs since ancient times and they were able to recognize their different features and uses. As a result, they were able to extract the active ingredients for use in remedies. These findings are the fruits of many years of experimentation and struggles to survive. Since then, herbs have been the main source of many medicines, until today.

Herbs are used in the human being's daily food and drink, such as pepper, spices, cumin and so on. Some of these are bitter, spicy, or sweet; some have pleasant odors and others have unpleasant odors.

Allāh ta'ālā (﷾) has bestowed many secrets in plants and herbs that serve humankind. Some of these help heal the human body and others corrupt it. Therefore, human beings are in a continuous search for these secrets throughout their lives, for these plants are a primary resource for living a healthy and satisfactory life.

As some herbs are toxic to human beings, some are also harmful and even deadly to jinn. Our focus is on the herbs that affect the jinn that violate human beings, either through dark magic or shaytānic possession. The following plants are very useful against jinn; they can hurt them and sometimes lead to their total destruction.

Ferula asafoetida (Angedan)

This plant has many names in different countries. It is extracted from the angedan tree and it is a glue (stinking gum) that has a very bitter taste; it is very spicy and dry. However, it has many medicinal uses. It treats gout, joint pain, parasites and worms, wounds, hemorrhoids, cough and gastrointestinal gas. It sharpens the vision, purifies the blood, reduces weight and melts fat, heals fevers and sciatica, dissolves chronic tumors and improves sexual ability.

Angedan's distinctive smell affects the jinn, whether they are inside or outside the human body. It suffocates them when you smell or swallow angedan. Therefore, it is advised to inhale an angedan steam every day. When swallowing it, do not exceed 1 gram in each swallow. It is a stomach softener and it helps reduce weight; it does not cause weight gain, as many people believe. Angedan should be preserved in a clay jar to help it maintain its essences for as long as possible.

Saffron
Saffron is a plant of the onion family that consists of delicate filaments. It is a yellowish color. Saffron is its common name known in most languages and it originated in Spain (Andalusia). It is planted today in many other countries. Saffron has a very refreshing smell and it is said in the prophetic sayings that saffron is Heaven's palm trees. It is usually planted in colder climates and the best saffron is planted in Spain. It is used to spice rice and beverages like tea and coffee, as well being used in ink to write the Qur'ān. Dragon blood tree powder (Dracaena cinnabari) is also used for this.

Saffron is known for strengthening the heart and clearing the eyes. It is also famous for its capacity to enhance sexual ability and generate urine. In addition, it affects the disbelieving, harmful jinn.

Olive Tree
Allāh ta'ālā (ﷻ) says in sūratu-n-nūr:

يوقد من شجرة مباركة زيتونة لا شرقية ولا غربية يكاد زيتها يضيء ولو لم تمسسه نار نور على نور يهدي الله لنوره من يشاء ويضرب الله الأمثال للناس والله بكل شيء عليم

"...fueled from a blessed olive tree, from neither the east nor the west,
whose oil almost gives light even when no fire touches it
—light upon light—
Allāh guides whomever He wills to His light;
Allāh draws such comparisons for people;
Allāh has full knowledge of everything." (24:35)

Therefore, the olive tree is one of the greatest and the most blessed of all plants by Allāh (ﷻ). Allāh ta'ālā (ﷻ) has mentioned this tree many times, as He did in sūratu-t-tin:

والتين والزيتون

"By the fig and the olive." (95:1)

Olives are known for being squeezed for their juice and their oil. The features of olives are many, one of which is that it is very beneficial for the stomach, either eaten or drunk. Olive oil is the best of oils and it is also used to strengthen the hair and detoxify the body.

Olive oil is most significant in the treatment of shaytānic possession and magic. By applying olive oil directly to the body, by adding it to water that has had Qur'ān recited over it, or by drinking it, the magic and possession will be invalidated.

Black Seed (Nigella sativa)
It has many names, such as: black cumin, Indian cumin, and "the blessed seed." Also, it has numerous benefits, as relayed in the prophetic saying, "It is a cure for every disease," or as the Prophet Muḥammad (ﷺ), may the peace and blessings of Allāh (ﷻ) upon him, said, "There is healing in black seed for all diseases except death." (Bukhārī 71:592)

Black seed is very beneficial in the treatment of almost all diseases, for it strengthens the immune system. Adding black seed powder to honey and olive oil is a mixture that, if taken three times a day, will prevent any illness from ever harming you.

Black seed is not beneficial for healthy people, but it is beneficial for sick people who suffer from certain diseases. People who are healthy may be harmed if they consume this herb, for it kills effective stomach and intestinal bacteria, which are very important for the digestive system's ability to absorb nutrients and decompose food.

Using black seed with olive oil together generates a very powerful treatment against shayṭānic possession and magic. It is also helpful to recite some Qur'ānic verses of protection. This heals, in particular, the type of possession that occurs during eating and drinking (through the mouth). This remedy repairs what has been damaged in the stomach from the magic and possession, as well as providing strength and protection against the assaulting jinn.

Apply black seed oil to the body, morning and evening, after reciting the Qur'ān (the protection verses and those that invalidate magic). This should be continued during and after the treatment.

Common Rue (Ruta graveolen)

It is also called "herb of grace" and "the jinn herb." There are two types: native and wild. It has green solid branches with jasmine flowers on them, which add a beautiful fragrance.

Ibn Bittar (ﷺ) mentions in his book to crush rue and mix it with honey. If a woman uses it as a suppository (with wool), it will warm the uterus, improve it and help her get pregnant, even if she is barren. It is one of the remedies that has been tested and has produced successful results, inshā'a-llāh (ﷻ).

Sniffing it empowers the inactive and weak brain, eliminates headaches, unblocks the vessels of the brain, purifies the head from waste and generates urine.

References

Qur'ān and Ḥadīth

- The Holy Qur'ān
- Ḥadīth of the Prophet Muḥammad (ﷺ) from the collections of Aḥmad, al-Tirmidhī, al-Bukhārī, Muslim, ibn Mājah, Abū Dāwūd and other canonical ḥadīth collections.

Classical Islamic medical literature

- Ibn Qayyim al-Jawziyya's *aṭ-Ṭibb al-nabawī*, available in several English translations, including the Islamic Texts Society's *Medicine of the Prophet*.
- ʿAbd al-Jabbār Ibn Sīnā's *al-Qānūn fī-l-ṭibb*, a medical and philosophical encyclopedia that has never been translated in its entirety. The introduction and conclusion are published in English by Brigham Young University as *The Physics of the Medicine* and *The Metaphysics of the Medicine*.
- Dāwūd al-Antāki's *Tadhkirat 'uli-l-albāb wa-l-jāmiʿa li-l-ajābu-l-ʿujāb* was a medical book that but it was popularly known as *Tadhkirat Dāwūd al-Antāki* or *Tadhkira*. It has not been translated into English yet.

Contemporary Arabic works

- ʿAbd al-Laṭīf ʿĀshūr, *al-Tadāwī bi-l-aʿshāb* (*The Medicinal Use of Herbs*).
- Faysal ibn Muḥammad ʿIrāqī, *al-Aʿshāb dawāʾ li-kull dāʾ* (*Herbs for Every Illness*).

Index

A

abdominal
  cramps, 51, 75, 86, 160
  pain, 81, 86
  swelling, 166
abscesses, 60, 155, 162
acacia, 136
acetic acid, 5
achilles plant, 65
acid reflux, 75 *See Also* Heartburn, Gastrointestinal Disorders
acidosis, 91
acne, 61, 69, 85, 89, 90, 92
Addison's disease, 136
adrenals, 88, 136
Aʿfiya, 39
aging, premature, 158
AIDS, 56
ʿĀʾisha (ﷺ), 17, 36, 119, 120
Ajlani, 39
Al-Baydawī, 35
Al-Bayhaqī, 131
al-manjam, 42
Al-Rabīʿ bin Haytham, 36
albumin, excess, 142
alchemilla, 64
ʿAlī (ﷺ), 192
alkaline minerals, 27
allergies, 5, 44
  infections, 147
  skin, 5
almonds, 25, 79
alopecia, 12, 106, 140, See also *Hair Loss*
  from infection, 12, 68
alpine, 53
aluminum, 5
amber, 11, 16, 77, 137, 181, 184, 188
  oil, 52, 181, 183, 184
ambergris, **137**
ammi, **106**
  roots, 106
ammonia, 15, 98
amoebiasis, 51, 75
  See also *Parasites, Worms*
amylase yeast, 5
anal ulcers, 98
analgesic substances, 112
Anas ibn Malik, 19, 20
anemia, 27, 34, 40, 48, 123, 132, 140, 158
angedan, **193-194**
angina, 65, 66, 111, 112
anise, 67, 74, 79, 160
  seeds, 180
  tea, 179
anti-aging, 25
antibacterial medications, 41
antibiotics, 5, 36, 39
  in tamarind, 91
antimony, 24
antispasmodic, 159
appetite stimulant, 104, 108, 122, 163
appetite, poor, 78, 134
apple cider vinegar, 54, 58, 68, 80
arak tree, 117, 118
arrhythmia, 11, 30
arteries
  blocked, 123, 163
  clear, 122
  softening, 26

arteriosclerosis, 31, 47, 56, 88, 103, 107, 129, 149, 159

arthritis, 93, 100, 103, 107, 113, 114, 116, 128, 140, 157, 169

arugula, 67, 92, 179, 187, 188
   juice, 67, 74, 92, 179, 187

asafetida, 71

ascites, 12, 62

asthenopia, 111

asthma, 11, 25, 29, 57, 77, 106, 111, 122, 135, 144, 169

Aswan, 37

at-Tadhkīra, 130

atherosclerosis, 140

āyātu-l-kursī, 172

B

back pain, 108, 116, 175

bacterial gastrointestinal infections, 100

bad breath, 9, 159

baldness, 44
   See also *Alopecia*

balsamic oil, 159

banalol, 159

bananas, 34, **44–49**

barley, 4, 51, **119–21**, 160
   extract, 120
   flour, 80
   flour poultice, 121
   juice, 119
   sugar, 4
   water, 51, 119, 120

bed bug rash, 81

bees
   act upon revelation, 3
   glue, 10
   stings, 6
   wax, 7, 9, 81

benzoic acid, 137, 144

better thinking, 47

bile
   acids, 140
   excess, 116
   lack of, 123

biotin, *See* Vitamin B₇

bites, 24
   poisonous, 95

black bread, 150

black lime, 82

black seed, 12, 15, 50, 63, 65, **67–78**, 81, 85, 176, 177, 184, 185, 189, 190, 195, 196
   and olive oil poultice, 71, 73
   oil, 12, 60, 67, 68, 69, 70, 71, 72, 73, 74, 75, 76, 77, 78, 81, 176, 177, 196

black tea, **124–25**

blackheads, 167

bladder
   infections, 110, 120, 143
   pain, 96, 110, 122
   stones, 111, 128, 143, 158
   ulcers, 47, 135

bleeding
   stomach, 29
   stops, 40, 41, 44

blisters, 6, 45, 154

bloating, 130, 131, 160

blonde hair lightener, 87

blood
   crusted, 172
   detoxifier, 91, 149
   excessive, 172
   purifier, 110, 194
   toxic, 172
   pressure, 51, 110, 149
      See Also hypertension and hypotension

purifier, 136, 166
sugar, reduces, 89, 92-3, 158
vessels, dilates, 106
renewal of, 92
body odor, 104, 109
body temperature,
    high, 91, 99, 119
    low, 83
body tissue
    sterilizes and strengthens,
        157
bones
    broken 59, 70, 110
boswellia carteri, 9, 12
bowel movements,
    lazy, 82
    to empty, 84
    weak, 107
brain, 25, 46, 117, 137, 144, 151,
    178, 185
    empowers, 196
    stroke, 32
breast
    feeding, 23, 47, 98, 160, 161
    inflammation, 160, 161
    milk, 41
        generates, 88, 98, 122, 140,
        160-1, 179
    pain, 100
breath, shortness of, 97, 106
breathing
    facilitates, 169
broad beans, 122, 131, **143**
broken bones, 59, 70, 110
bronchitis, 111
    chronic, 137
bruises, 70
bruising, 59
Burni dates, 19, 21

burns, 6, 83, 98, 104, 130, 142,
    155

C

cabbage, 62, 71, **157–58**, 157,
    158
    root, 71
    seeds, 62
caffeine, 124, 152, 153
    overdose, 124
caffeoyl, 152
calcium, 4, 40, 88, 89, 93, 107,
    120, 122, 123, 125, 126, 129,
    135, 140, 142, 150, 158, 164
    oxalate, 136
calf kidneys, 85
Caliph ar-Rashīd, 192
calluses, 12, 128
camel's milk, 76, 177, 185, 187
cancer, 5, 15, 23, 37, 53, 77, 130
    anti-cancer, 53
    colon, 27
    colorectal, 32
    malignant, 10
    skin, 61
    sores, 60
    prevention, 23
carbohydrates, 20, 21, 23, 26,
    33, 39, 41, 45, 107, 110, 123,
    128, 131, 152, 158, 164, 190
carnation, 8, 74, 144, **147–48**,
    187
    oil, 148
carob, **99**
carotid arteries, 171, 172, 174
carrots
    juice, 11, 15, 25, 75, 77, 93
    seeds, 188
    yellow, **93–94**

castor
  beans, **100**
  leaves, 100
  oil, 54, 76, 100, 101
catalase, 5
cataracts, 64
cauliflower, **146**
cavities, 46, 117, 132, 146
celery, 85, 126, 187, 188
cellulose, 21, 41, 89, 128, 150
cerebral cortex, 153
cerebral palsy, 103
cerebrospinal gland extract, 89
chameleon leather, 69
chamomile, 25, 29, 68, **86–87,**
  177
  poultice, 87
  steam, 87
  tea, 25, 29, 68
cheese, 58, 62, 63, 64, 65, 75,
  131, 132
chest
  pain, 44, 84, 96, 106, 111, 126,
  133
  stuffy, 163
chicken gallbladder, 188
chickpeas, **97**, 185, 188
chilblains, 61
child development, 46
childbirth, 14, 20, 41, 68, 177–
  81, 179
  increases contractions, 89
chlorate, 164
chlorine, 5, 40
chlorophyll, 142, 158
chlorophyllin, 144
cholera, 21, 53, 164
cholesterol, 47, 50, 129
choline, 26
chromium, 5

chymus, 140
cinnamic acid, 139
cinnamic aldehyde, 145
cinnamon, **144–45,** 181, 185
circulation
  cleanser, 149
  poor, 102, 115
  strengthens, 151
citric acid, 5, 91, 165
citrine, 164
citron, 163
cloves, 50, 51, 52, 53, 54, 55, 56,
  61, 67, 71, 76, 186, 189
coconuts, 47
coffee, 132, **152–53**
  beans, 24, 31, 152
  fruit, 152
  tree, 152
colds,
  chronic, 139
  common, 53, 64, 73, 85, 87,
  97, 99, 112, 113, 115, 122, 130,
  139, 140, 144, 160
  mild, 150
colic, 74, 163 *See Also* Intestinal
colon *See Also* Intestinal
  obstruction, 130
  pain, 75
Commiphora molmol, 71, 73
common beans, 122, **142**
common mallow. *See* Mallow
congestive hepatopathy, 111
conjunctivitis, 87, 111, 130
connective tissue pain, 12,
  See *Rheumatism*
constipation, 8, 24, 32, 34, 41,
  74, 82, 91, 95-6, 99, 100, 105,
  107, 109, 116, 123, 124, 128,
  132, 136, 146, 150, 153, 155,
  166

chronic, 48, 104
with painful cramps, 155
prevented by dates, 21
severe, 82
copper, 5, 30, 107, 123, 158
coriander, 64, 83, 154, **159**
cornea, inflamed, 84
coronet, 130
cosmetics, 5, 69, 114, 116, 123,
167
cough, 29, 30, 61, 44, 62, 65, 90,
96, 98, 105, 111, 112, 115, 119,
122, 130, 135, 139, 140, 144,
150, 161, 169, 193
at night, 167
bloody, 126
dry, 135
chronic, 84, 133, 167
dry, 155
cramps
Also See *Abdominal Cramps*
prevent, 169
cryptitis, 90
CSSI, 100, 104, 113
cucumbers, **109**
cumin, 50, 74, 160, 166, 178
cupping. *See* ḥijāma
cuts, 6

D

dandruff, 54
date molasses, 25, 29, **30**, 31
date palm, 17, 18, 19, 33, 36, 39
location of, 37
pollen, **126–27**, 189
shoots, **89**
seeds, **31**, 37
dates, **17–43**, 59, 65, 84, 126
3 types of, 39

Burni, 19
childbirth, 20, 35
during nifās, 18
in the Quran, 17
postpartum, 36
rubbing on newborns' lips,
18, 23
sunna of eating 7, 24
Dāwūd Al-Anṭākī, 130, 133, 135,
140, 154, 161, 163, 169
deafness, 160
accident or infection, 52
dental erosion, 163
dermatitis, 35, 81, 86, 98, 121,
146, 150
detoxifier, powerful, 92
deuterium, 5
dextrin, 153
dextrose, 4
diabetes, 31, 48, 62, 70, 89, 90,
92, 93, 99, 123, 126, 127, 134,
142, 158, 162, 175
diarrhea, 7, 29, 35, 41, 45, 47,
74, 86, 90, 93, 94, 111, 118,
121, 126, 144, 148, 153, 159
chronic, 93, 150
infant and toddler, 93
digestion
helps, 144, 160
digestive
bleeding, 165
disorders, 21, 48, 90, 99, 149,
158
juices
stimulant, 108, 151, 159
system, activates, 94, 143
dill, 85
juice, 9
diphtheria, 52, 62, 66, 140, 161
diuresis, 84, 157

diuretic, 51
diverticulitis, 46
dizziness, 27, 55, 64, 67, 68, 163, 175
doum, **110**
Dr. Amīn Ruwīhā, 154
Dr. Fania, 151
Dr. Heige, 132
Dracaena cinnabari, 194
dragon blood tree powder, 194
drooling, prevents, 160
dropsy, 72, 93, 123, 130, 140, 147
drug side-effects, 153
dyer's broom, 65
dysentery, 51, 112, 121
dyspepsia, 51, 137

E

ear
    ache, 67
    diseases, 12, 63, 160
    infection, 140
    pain, 12, 172
eczema, 61, 87, 93
    chronic, 112
edema, 34, 48
efficiency during exams, 42
eggs, 5, 25, 55, 69, 77, 146, 187, 189
    shells, 72
    whites, 130, 155, 167
    yolks, 81, 114, 144, 186, 187
Egypt, 37, 39, 118, 119, 131, 154
endocrine diseases, 69
enema, 65, 111, 122, 154, 160
energy, increase, 47, 66, 82
enteritis, 121, 123, 128
entero-colitis, 86

epilepsy, 7, 81, 94, 96
epistaxis, 160
erectile dysfunction.
    See Impotence
essential alkaloids, 120
essential oils, 112, 131, 139, 141, 144, 154
eucalyptus oil, 12, 59
exercise, 64
exhaustion, 48
eye
    beautifies, 135
    diseases, 7, 24, 56, 64, 75, 130, 171
    infection, 88
    pain, 172, 175
    strain, 111
    See Also Vision
eyeliner, 7, 147

F

face
    brightens, 160
    cleanser, 167
    mask, 167
    problems, 174
Fajr
    don't go back to sleep, 78
fatigue, 34, 48, 92, 142, 148, 158, 161, 165
fats, 26, 39, 91, 128, 131
    melts, 194
favus, 101
female reproductive system, 147 *See Also* Uterus and Ovaries
fennel, 63, 65, 76, 83, **122**
    steam, 122

fenugreek, 14, 61, 73, 76-7, 79, 80, **96**, 154, 157, 177-8
   seeds, 96
Ferula asafoetida, 71, 193
fever, 73, 90, 91, 109, 110, 111, 116, 119, 126, 130, 135, 150, 153, 170, 194
   caused by abdominal diseases, 91
figs, 24, **79–85**
   leaves, 85
   "milk", 80
   tree sap, 81
   wood, 80
fish, 25, 42, 69, 126
flax seed, **154–56**
   oil, 92, 155
   poultice, 154
flower oil, 5, 69, 140, 159
flu, 9, 52, 64, 95, 96, 126
fluid production, 122
fluoride, 129
folic acid, 4
food poisoning, 163
foot calluses, 12
foot pain, 174
forgetfulness, 171
formic acid, 5
freckles, 44, 88, 144, 150, 161, 163
fructose, 4, 24
fruit, 132
   juice, 64, 88

G

galangal, **108**, 188
gallbladder
   diseases, 73, 128, 132, 170
   infections, 126

   pain, 106
   stones, 27, 54, 73, 89, 97, 104, 116, 155, 161
gangrene, 10, 116
garden cress, 71, 184
garlic, 7, 30, 31, **50–56**, 68, 71, 75, 76, 186, 189
   bread, 53
   odor, remove, 55, 159
   steam, 50-53
gas (gastro-intestinal) 47, 51, 75, 94, 95, 103, 108, 111, 115, 122, 133, 140, 147, 159, 160, 161, 162, 163, 164, 169, 193
gastric
   acid, 27
   acidity, 7, 44, 45, 128, 169
   bleeding, 29
   cramps, 142
   mucus membranes, 169
   ulcers, 27, 77, 86, 96, 102, 150
gastro-colic response, 79
gastro-enteritis, 95, 96, 99
gastrointestinal
   bleeding, 149
   colic, 155
   disorders, 45, 170
   infections, 100, 155
   muscle spasms, 106
   ulcers, 136, 158, 165
   weakness, 120
Genista tinctoria, 65
ghee, 186, 187, 188
ginger, 11, 44, **115**, 181, 185, 188
ginger tea, 115
gingivitis, 80, 95, 113
glandular function, 150
gluconic acid, 5
glucose, 39, 118, 150
glycerin, 129, 135, 166, 167

goat scybala, 83
goat's milk, 184
gourd seeds, 76
gout, 42, 81, 102, 104, 107, 140,
    157, 164, 193
grape
    leaves, 180
    sugar, 118
green beans.
    See Common Beans
grilled onions, 59
growth hormone deficiency,
    142
gums, 10, 54, 92, 95, 118, 147,
    169
    bleeding, 113, 116, 118
    healthy, 129
    infections, 114
    sore, 10
gynecological disorders, 68, 99,
    177–81
    prevent, 177

H

hair
    dye, 114
    fragile, 92, 101
    lightener, 87
    loss, 12, 44, 63, 67, 92, 116,
    140, *See also Alopecia*
    strengthener, 149, 151
Ḥajj, 176
halitosis, 9
hallucinations, 45
    prevents, 159
headaches, 47, 55, 61, 67, 87,
    100, 102, 107, 109, 122, 124,
    147, 154, 159, 163-4, 171-2,
    174-6, 196

heart
    arrhythmia, 11, 30
    diseases, 26, 74, 142
    muscle, inflammation, 11
    pressure, 11
    rate, low, 124
    stimulant, 144, 147
    strengthens, 26, 114, 159, 169
    vulnerable, 66
    weak, 11, 102-3, 149
heartburn, prevents, 159
    Also See *Acid Reflux*
heavy hydrogen, 5
heels, cracked, 81
hemoglobin, 158
hemorrhoids, 21, 32, 85, 96, 98,
    116, 123, 130, 133, 135, 149,
    193
    bleeding, 28
henna, 29, 69
hepatitis, 72, 88, 93, 97, 106
herpes, 9, 68, 95, 140, 142
hibiscus flower, 13
hiccups, 160, 169
ḥijāma, **171–76**
Hippocrates, 119
hoarse voice, 9
honey, **3–16**, 27-9, 44, 50-1, 53,
    56-60, 62-78, 81, 83-4, 89, 94,
    96-7, 99, 111, 130, 139-140,
    144, 146, 150, 154-5, 160-1,
    165-6, 169, 176-7, 181, 183-
    190, 195-6
    carries medical extracts, 3
hordenine, 120, 121
hormones, 5
hormones, sex, 89
hydropsy, 48

hypertension, 32-3, 45, 47, 51, 56, 71, 89, 103, 110, 127, 142, 149, 159
hypotension, 65

I

Ibn ʿAbbās, 3
Ibn al-Qayyim, 131, 172
Ibn Bittar, 196
Ibn Isḥāq, 131
Ibn Mājah, 4, 119, 171
Ibn Mubārak, 131
Ibn Nawāwi, 17
Ibn-Sīnā, 135, 140, 157
Imām Aḥmad bin Ḥanbal, 171
immune system
    function, 134
    protects, 151
    strengthens, 157, 158, 165, 195
impotence, 77, 90, 96, 104, 175, **182–91**
    cause of, 184
indigestion, 47, 65, 92, 100, 108, 109, 113, 115, 123-4, 136, 140, 142-3, 147, 151, 159, 163
infections, 98, 100
    cure, 169
infertility, 15, 27, 76
    See Also Reproductive Organs
    Allah's will, 182
    egg fertilization, 178
    female, 89, 177
    male, 186, 190
    male and female, 104
inflammation, 26, 44, 45, 48, 62, 81, 82, 90, 155, 163
    of the nerves, 48
influenza, 9

injury, 6
inositol, 142
insanity, 6, 28, 45
insect repellant, 109, 133
insomnia, 6, *See also* Sleeping Disorders
intestinal
    bacterial overgrowth, 140
    cleanser, 154
    colic, 151, 170
    disorders, 86, 91
    pain, 75, 122, 133
    ulcers, 156
    weak, 132
invertase yeast, 5
iodine, 4, 140, 150, 158, 159
iron, 4, 27, 30, 34, 37, 40, 88, 107, 109, 120, 122-3, 125-6, 140, 142, 150, 157-8, 164
irregular heartbeat, *See* heart rate
irritability, 40, 45, 137
ischemia, 44
itchiness, 44, 83, 130, 159, 163
itchy scalp, 44

J

jaundice, 44, 47, 97, 123, 143, 157
jaw pain, 55
jinn, 172, 173, 175, 193, 194, 196
joint pain, 12, 174, 193, *See Also* Rheumatism
juniper, **133–34**

K

kidney

diseases, 32, 47, 48, 62, 128, 132-3
  failure, prevent, 26
  health, 88
  infections, 26, 71, 120, 143
  inflammation, 26
  lean, 44
  pain, 143-4
  stones, 13, 26-7, 62, 71, 88-9, 92, 94, 97, 123, 140, 143, 146, 155-6
  tumors, 83
  ulcers, 44, 135
  weakness, 97, 147
King's Malady, 164
King's Paste, 188
knees, swelling 174
kohl, 7, 24

L

lā 'ilāha 'illa-llāh, 173
labor, *See* Childbirth
lactic acid, 5
lady's mantle, 64
laxative, 91, 97, 107, 123, 154, 161
laziness, 25, 78, 91
lazy bowels, 82
lead, 5
leg stiffness, 175
lemon, 65, 71, **163–68**
  balm, 86
  brine, 164
  flower petals, 163
  juice, 44, 51-4, 58, 73, **163-68**
  oil, 164
  peel, 71, 164
  seeds, 164

lenolic acid, 89
lentils, **130–32**
leprosy, 15, 69, 130
lethargy, 25, 78
lettuce, **103–5**
leukocytes, 142
libido, 15
licorice, 75, **135–36**
  root, 75, 135-36
  root juice, 135
lifespan
  prolongs, 137
lime, black, 82
lithium, 5
liver
  cleans, 146
  enhances, 169
  strengthens, 142
  diseases, 13, 94-5, 132, 140-42 *See Also* Hepatitis
  function, 160
  infections, 72, 154, 166
  pain, 135
  protects, 165
  reactivates, 104
  spasms, 140
  strengthens, 94
  vessels, unblocks, 144
  weakness, 97, 113
lung
  coughing up blood, 126
  cleans, 144, 161
  clears, 140
  congestion, 102
  diseases 8, 24, 30, 44, 47, 73, 79, 97, 120, 135, 140, *See Also* Respiratory System
  infections, 102, 154
  pain, 130
  phlegm, 92, 94, 100

tonic, 97
lupin, 89
  juice, 157
  oil, 89
lymph node
  adenitis, 155
  infection, 155
lymphatic system, blocks, 130

M

magic, 172-73, 193, 195-96
magnesium, 4, 23, 33-5, 135, 150
male sexual health, **182–91**
malic acid, 165
mallow, **98**
malnutrition, 45, 47, 190-91
manganese, 5, 140
mango, 5, 25, 69
Mao, 39
Maryam, 18, 35-6
  dates, 19, 42
mastitis, 160-61, 169
measles, 47, 90, 155
meat, 132
meditation, 47
melon, **123**
memorization, faster, 78
memory, 54, 79
meningitis, 73
menopause, 14
menstrual blood
  generates, 180
menstrual cycle, 122
  regulates, 85, 127
  pain, 85, 88, 92, 97, 111, 144, 157, 170, 180, 181
mental
  activation, 78

illness, 6, 28, 41, 81
menthol, 169
microalbuminuria, 46
migraines, 45, 87, 175
milk, hot, 8, 51, 52, 67
minerals, 128
mouth
  and tongue ulcers, 159
  cleanser, 66
  inflammation, 11
  moldiness in the, 164
  rash, 164
  ulcers, 83, 86
mucus membranes, irritates, 160
multiengine, 120
muscle
  activates, 165
  building, 55
  spasms, gastrointestinal, 106
musk, 173, 180
mustard, **102–3**
  foam, 83
  118, 187
  seeds, 103, 187
mutton, 58
myocarditis, 11
myrosin, 118
myrrh, 71, 76, 187

N

nasal congestion, 87
nausea, 8, 74, 94, 104, 163, 169
nephrolithiasis, 13
nerve pain, 86
nerves
  inflammation of, 48
  soothes, 142, 149

nervous system, 26, 40, 46, 52,
93-4, 104, 137, 147, 151, 153,
163
activating to, 114, 153
calms and strengthens, 52
calms, 169
exhaustion, 112
regulation, 46
relax, 75
sexual dysfunction, 185
tranquilizer, 113
neurasthenia, 89, 112
neurological
disorders, 109
spasms, 114
niacin, See Vitamin B₃
nickel, 5
nicotinic acid, 4, 33, 35
nifās, 18, 41, 175
night blindness, 27
nose
disorders, 171
pain, 172
bleed, 149, 166
numbness, 45
nutmeg, 94
nyctalopia, 27

oil, 6, 11-2, 51-2, 54-6, 58-63,
67, 69, 76, 80-2, 116, 133, 178,
185, 189, 195-6
oil and black seed poultice,
71, 73
tree, 195
onion, **57–66**, 92, 190
juice, 57-61, 63-5, 186-7, 190
odor, removes, 159
poultice, 57-8, 60, 63-5
soup, 59, 62
steam, 59, 64
ophthalmia, 56
ophthamology, 7 See Also Eyes
and Vision
orange juice, 52, 78
orchitis, 160
organic acids, 107
organs
strengthens, 137
ospargen, 135
ovaries
stimulates, 127
oxalic acid, 5
oxygen absorption enhanced,
158
oxytocin, 41

O

oak bark, 13
obesity, 47-8, 132, 142, 161, 166
obsession, 81
oleic acid, 153
oliban, 9, 12, 185, 186
oligochaetes, 111
oligospermia, 184
olive, 98, **116**
leaf, 116

P

painkiller, 116, 122, 148
palm acacia, 27
palm fronds, 27
palm tree pollen, **29**, 190
palmitic acid, 153
palpitations, 83
prevents, 159
parasites, 22, 37, 53-4, 65, 76,
90-1, 93, 99, 106, 112, 122,
146, 157-8, 160, 164-5, 169,

193, *See also Worms,*
  Amoebiasis
Parkinson's disease, 157
parotitis, 155
parsley, 54-5, **88**
peaches, **107**
pear juice, 51, 75
peas, 131
Pedanius Dioscorides, 157, 161
Pellagra, 35, 45, 164
pepper, 154
peppermint, 78, **169–70**
Peptic Ulcer Disease, 47
perforated ulcers, 8
periodontitis, 95
peristalsis, 24
peroxide, 5
pertussis, *See Also* Whooping
  Cough 29
pharyngitis, 82
phlegm, 92
  excess, 44
phosphatase, 5
phosphate, 135
phosphorus, 4, 25-6, 37, 42, 88-
  9, 107, 120, 122-3, 126, 129,
  142, 146, 150, 158
phrethrum, 188
pine seeds, 25, 188
pistachio, 79, 190
plague, 56
pneumonia, 57
poisoning, 16, 24, 50, 79, 153,
  163, 171
pomegranate, 77
  peel, 11, 83
  powder, 71
possession. *See* Shayṭānic
  possession
postpartum, *See* Childbirth

potassium, 4, 32-4, 45, 48, 107,
  109, 120, 122-3, 135, 142, 150,
  164
potatoes, 34, 161
prayers, do them, 77
pregnancy, 41, 47, 142, 144,
  147, 175, 178
prickly pear fruit, 72
Prophet Muḥammad, 3-4, 7-8,
  17-19, 20-1, 23-4, 36, 67, 74,
  117, 119-20, 131, 171-72, 176,
  195
prostate
  disease, 58
  health, 76
  prostatitis, 16
protein, 37, 46, 49, 89, 126, 127,
  131, 152
psoriasis, 27, 95, 106 *See Also*
  Skin Disorders
psychological diseases, 59
pus, 60
pyroglutamic acid, 5

Q

quince, 130
Qur'ān, 3, 7, 17, 42, 64, 77, 126,
  130, 173, 192, 194--97
Qur'ānic water, 173

R

rabbit
  gallbladder, 178
  rennet, 178
radish, 8, 15, 58, 76, **140–41**,
  177, 188, 190
  juice, 8, 140

roots, 140
seeds, 15, 58, 76, 177, 188, 190
relaxation, 41
renal colic, 13, 106, 149
reproductive enhancement, 15, 25, 58 See Also Infertility
reproductive organs, See Also Infertility
  strengthens, 151
  diseases, 158
respiratory
  analgesic, 155
  conditions, 82, See Also Lung diseases
  phlegm, 92, 94, 100
  tonic, 114
rheumatism, 12, 24, 48, 59, 70, 81, 86, 94, 99, 100, 103, 107, 113, 128, 133-34, 150, 164, 169, 174
rheumatoid arthritis, 92
rhinitis, 115
rhinoceros horn
  filings, 15
  powder, 190
riboflavin, See Vitamin B$_2$

rose
  petals, 92
  syrup, 11
  water, 90, 117, 179, 180, 181
royal jelly, 11-2, 15-6, 69, 189
rue, 79, 81, 184, 196
runny nose, 163

S

saffron, **113–14**, 173, **179-81**, 194

flowers, 113
oil, 113
ṣalāh, 173
Sālim ibn Sālim, 131
saliva production, 115
Salmān bin ʿAmr, 20
sandfish skink, 188
sap, sweetgum, 139
scabies, 54, 87, 89, 97, 100
scalp, 168
schistosomiasis, 75, 90, 106
sciatica, 108, 116, 140, 194
sclerosis, 47
scorpion bite, 95
scurvy, 47, 48, 163
sea urchin skin, 73
secretin, 149
sedative, 105
seizures, 94, 96
semen, See Also Infertility, male
  lack of, 183
  production, 154
senna, 136
sesame oil, 16, 44, 61, 69, 130
sex hormones, 135
sexual (male)
  ability, improves, 55, 89, 114, 126, 137, 140, 154, 161, 170, 185
  desire, 15, 47
  dysfunction (male), **182–91**
  glands, 89, 122
  vitality, increase, 97
shayṭānic possession, 172, 193 195-96
sheep's milk, 108, 186
shortness of breath, 175
shoulder pain, 171, 172, 174
silicon, 5, 109
sinigirin, 118

siwak, 10, **117–18**
skeleton, strengthens, 151
skin *See Also* Sores and Wounds
   allergies, 5
   blackheads, 167
   blemishes, 88, 100
   cancer, 61
   clarity, 5
   diseases, 15, 69, 80, 89, 94-5,
   140, 155, 162
      chronic, 133
   facial cleanser, 167
   facial mask, 167
   flaking, 155
   infections, 142, 169
      chronic, 106
   pigmentations, 57, 140
   reddening, 101, 104
   soothes and moisturizes, 123
   spots, 163
   swelling, 98
   tumors, 104, 130, 161
      infected, 159
   ulcers, 10, 29, 51, 80, 87, 92,
   93, 95, 97, 140, 154
   cracking, 162
   dry, 123
   facial, 109
sleeping disorders, 6, 67, *See*
   Also Insomnia
smallpox, 83, 88
snail fever, 75
snake bite, 47, 95
sneezing, 115
soda ash, 79-80
sodium, 5, 33, 40, 45, 107, 150,
   158
sore throat, 82-3, 90, 96, 102-3,
   112, 115, 164, 171
sores, 29

cancerous, 60
chronic, 10
sperm
   generation, 44
   low sperm count, 184
   production, 47, 184
spiritual herbalism, **192–96**
spleen
   cleans, 146
   diseases, 73, 97, 114, 157
   enhances, 169
   infection, 154
   pain, 135
   tonic, 63
   strengthens, 94, 142
splenic flexure syndrome, 32
sprains, 88, 150
sputum, 30, 115, 117, 129, 135,
   139, 144
starch, 150
stercoral ulcers, 32
stinging nettle, 60, **149**
stings, 24
stomach
   ache, 114
   adds moisture to, 104
   bleeding, 29
   cleanser, 50, 84, 99, 147
   colic, 115
   diseases, 128
   gas, 51 *See Also* Gas
   gurgling, 130
   infections, 135
   moldiness, 128
   tonic, 114
   virus, 95
   weakness, 116
   softens, 47, 140
   stimulant, 144

strengthens, 139, 144, 147, 159
stomatitis, 11, 90, 102
Story of ʿAlī and Christian Physician, 192
strawberries, **89–90**, 92
strength, 82
    greater, 66
sucrose, 4, 126
Sufis, 152
sugar cane, 28, 57, 74, 75, 136, 159, 181, 183, 184
sugar
    reduces desire for, 159
sulfur, 4, 26, 107, 123, 136, 140, 150, 162
sunflower, **129**
    seeds, 129
sunna, 4, 174
sūratu-l-baqara, 173
sūratu-l-falaq, 172
sūratu-l-ḥashr, 173, 175
sūratu-l-ikhlāṣ, 172
sūratu-n-nās, 172
sweat
    excessive, 133
    generates, 139
    increases, 144
sweetgum, **139**
sycamore, **95**

T

tahnik, 23
talbīna, 120
tamarind, 91
tannins, 28, 112, 124, 125, 145, 153, 169
tea, **124–25**
temperature, low, 83

testicles, 76, 184
    inflammation, 160
testosterone, 127
tharīd, 119
thiamine, *See* Vitamin B$_1$
thirst, 84, 126, 135, 163
    excessive, 109
    prevents, 159
three deadly things, 14
throat pain, 172 *See Also* Sore Throat
thrombosis, 50, 66
thyme, 58-9, 61, 65, 73, 85, **111–12**, 126, 159, 160, 178
    oil, 112
thyroid, 88, 93, 151, 165
tiger nut sedges, 188
tin, 5
titanium, 5
tomato, 58, 75, **128**
    juice, 58
tongue
    diseases, 11
    infections, 164
tonic, general, 54
tonsillitis, 63, 86, 102, 111, 116
tooth
    abscessed, 83
    decay, 46, 146
    enamel damage, 165
    healthy, 129
    irritation, 41
    loss, 54
    pain, 55, 111, 147, 160, 169, 171, 174
    protect, 68
    strengthens, 10, 110, 151
toxicity, 50, 79, 133, 147, 163
trachea
    inflammation, 167

spasm, 106
rough, 44
soothes and cleans, 135
tracheitis, 82
trachoma, 56
tranquilizer, natural, 105, 122
tuberculosis, 11, 53, 92, 99, 120
tumors, 100, 146, 154
  chronic, 194
  infected, 154
  malignant, 10
  skin *See* Skin
  thick, 81
  visible, 83
turnip, white, 140, **161–62**
typhoid, 51, 112

U

ulcers, 8, 147
  anal, 98
  gastric, 27, 77, 86, 94, 96, 102, 136, 150
  intestinal, 156
  mouth, 83, 86
  mouth and throat, 90
  skin, 10, 29, 51, 80, 87, 92, 93, 95, 140, 154
underweight, 96
ureter spasm, 106
uric acid, 132, 146
urinary tract, 154
  cleanser, 26, 51
  diseases, 154, 158
  infection, 87
  pain, 155
  stones, 142
urine and urination
  and sperm generation, 44
  blood in, 110, 154

cleanses, 161
copious, 134
difficult or painful, 58, 72, 89, 92, 96-7, 99, 100, 110, 135
frequent, 109
generates, 104
involuntary, 72
thick, 135
painful, 88, 160
production, 114, 119, 123, 124, 129, 132, 140, 142, 143, 144, 149, 153, 154, 160, 169, 196
retention, 106, 107, 110, 113, 114, 126, 144, 160
urolithiasis, 142, 143, 158
uterus, 35, 36, 41, **177-79**
  astringes, 160
  diseases of, 144
  heat in, 180
  stimulant, 144
  warms, 147, 196

V

vaginal
  discharge, 81
  shower, 177
vanilla, 144
varicose veins, 10, 60
Vaseline, 5-6
vessels
  clears blockaes, 161
  unblocks, 140, 146
vinegar, 10, 11, 44, 61, 67, 69, 72, 78, 80, 96, 100, 104, 130, 140, 150, 159, 160, 161, 163, 169
vision, 94, 104, 114, 122

blurry, 147
clears, 144
sharpens, 193
visual impairments, 157
vitamin
    A, 4, 26, 42, 45, 88, 93, 107,
        109, 122, 128, 140, 142,
        150, 158
    B, 88, 109, 122, 126, 128, 142,
        150
    B$_1$ (thiamine), 4, 26, 33
    B$_2$ (riboflavin), 4, 26, 33, 142,
        164
    B$_3$ (niacin) 4, 33, 35, 45, 163
    B$_7$ (biotin), 4, 88
    B-complex, 4, 40, 45
    C, 40, 45, 48, 88, 107, 109,
        122-23, 126, 128, 140, 142,
        158, 163, 165
    D, 4, 128
    deficiency, 45
    K, 4
vitiligo, 15, 69, 80, 106, 140, 163
vocal cord
    disorders, 146, 157
    nodules, 144
    strain, 115
voice
    hoarse, 9
    clears, 135
vomiting, 8, 41, 45, 143, 144,
    148, 163, 170
    relieves, 41

W

walnuts, 79, 188
    leaves, 13
warts, 80, 100, 144

watermelon, 123
    juice, 44
    seeds, 44, 130
weakness, general, 34, 77, 120,
    134, 158, 163
weight loss, 64, 194
wheat, **150–51**
    bread, 169
    flour, 61, 69, 150
    juice, 58
white turnip. See Turnip, White
whooping cough, 29, 53, 57, 82,
    90, 106, 113
worms, 41, 53, 65, 76, 90, 93,
    107, 111, 112, 146, 157, 160,
    164, 165, 193, See also
    Parasites, Amoebiasis
wounds, 6, 29, 40, 44, 66, 93, 95,
    121, 130, 135, 139, 146, 157,
    168, 193
    chronic, 51
    contaminated, 149
    septic, 60
    sterilizer, 66, 148

Y

yellow carrot, 93
yogurt, 64, 71-2, 75, 77, 85, 97,
    99, 109, 120
youthfulness, 66

Z

Zād al-Miʿād fī Hadī Khayr al-
    ʿIbād, 4, 172
Zam-Zam water, 4
zinc, 5, 28, 40, 42

Index of Quotes from the Quran

A good tree whose root is firm and whose branches are high in the sky...(14:24-25), 19

Allāh (﷾) has control of the heavens and the earth. (42:49-50), 182

And, if you shake the trunk of the palm tree toward you (19:25-26), 20, 35

And your Lord inspired the bees saying...(16:68-69), 3

From the date palm come clusters of low-hanging dates...(6:99), 17

...fields, palm trees laden with fruit... (26:148), 126

Tall palm trees laden with clusters of dates. (50:10), 19, 126

With its fruits, its date palm trees with sheathed clusters...(55:11), 17

Index of Quotes from the Hadith

'Aʾis̲h̲a, a home which has no dates, has within it a hungry family, 17, 36

Among the trees, there is a tree, the leaves of which do not fall, 18

Break your fasting by eating dates, 18

Burni Dates are a remedy which do not bear a malady, 19

Dates are from Paradise and contain a cure for poison., 17

Feed your wives dates during their nifās, 18

He who eats seven dates as he awakens, no poison, 17, 36

He who licks three drops (of honey) every month, 4

Healing is by three (means): a drink of honey, 3, 171

I brought my newborn son to the Prophet (ﷺ) and He named him Ibrāhīm, 18

Ripe dates are from Paradise, 24

Take talbīna and have the patient sip it, 120

Talbīna soothes the heart of the patient, 120

The best dates are Burni dates, 19, 21

The highest date has the best cure, 19

The Prophet Muḥammad (ﷺ) used to break his fast before praying with some fresh dates..., 19, 20

The Prophet Muḥammad (ﷺ) used to prepare barley soup, 119

There is healing in black seed for all diseases except death, 67, 195

When one of you is fasting, he should break his fast with dates, 20

You should eat the beneficial thing that is unpleasant, 120

www.ingramcontent.com/pod-product-compliance
Lightning Source LLC
Chambersburg PA
CBHW070412270326
41926CB00014B/2791